BREATHE

BRAHMA SHAKTI

VINYASA YOGA

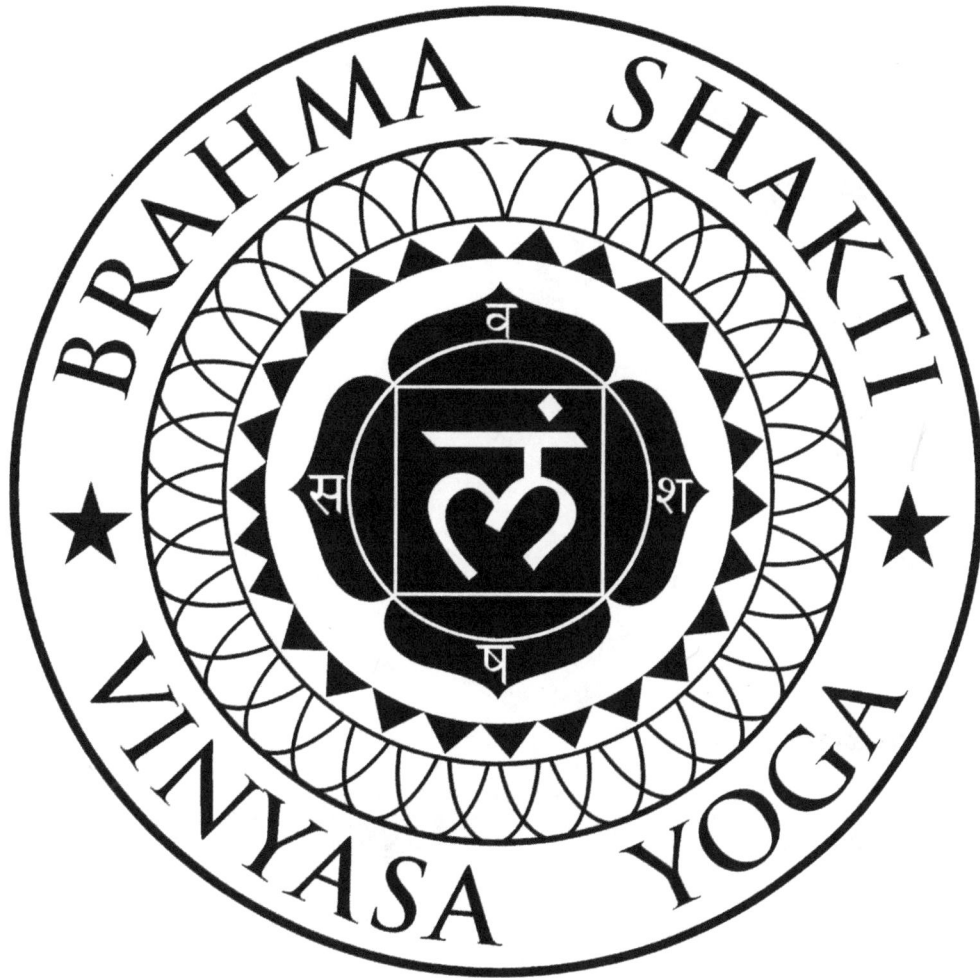

A SUSTAINABLE PRACTICE FOR LIFE
BORN FROM ASHTANGA YOGA

MARK FLINT . KPJAYI

BRAHMA SHAKTI VINYASA YOGA

First published in 2021 by Yorkshire Buddha
Text copyright Mark Flint 2019-2-14

Photography and edit credits to:
Photographs: Karolina Bratek.
Photographs edit: Elinor.
Text edit: Papa Joe Barfield.

Print ISBN: 978-0-9957560-6-9
e-Book ISBN: 978-0-9957560-7-6

Published by Yorkshire Buddha

DISCLAIMER

The views, opinions and advice given in this book are based on the personal experiences of the author, who is not a qualified mainstream health practitioner.

The author disclaims any liabilities or loss in connection with the exercises, diet and any other information or advice herein. If you have a persistent health problem you should consult a health practitioner.

Please be aware that not all yoga exercises are suitable for everyone straight away and it takes time to be able to complete all the asanas. When you have completed suryanamaskar A & B the author suggests you find a competent and qualified teacher to help you further with the series of asanas.

Dedicated to all the yogis past and present who have helped me develop this system

TABLE OF CONTENTS

FOREWORD

I wanted to share the vinyasa system in a way that it was suitable to both sexes, young and old, fat or thin, a practice for everyone, a practice for a lifetime where everyone could continue to practice maintaining the benefits.

BKS Iyengar practiced into his nineties, Krishnamacharya was still teaching at 100 years old, these were true yogis whose example we should all follow.

A note to teachers, do not teach just for money, teach from the heart as ones own Dharma.

"Practice what you preach"

SECTION 1: WHO. WHAT. WHY.

WHO - ABOUT THE AUTHOR

Mark Flint, was born in Britain, he started his career as a United Kingdom Professional Golfing Association (PGA) professional playing and teaching golf before joining his family automobile and real estate business in the UK.

After being diagnosed with rheumatoid arthritis at only 29 years old, he embarked on a course of self-discovery and healing through diet and yoga, rejecting the British doctors advice, which would have led to a lifetime of suppressing medicine.

Mark settled in Mysore in south India in 1999 where he learned the theory and practice of Hatha and Ashtanga Vinyasa Yoga.

Mark has authored 2 previous publications on yoga, *Yoga and Diet Cured my Arthritis* and *Parampara* an Ashtanga yoga practice manual.

His qualifications include:

- UK PGA Golf Professional

- Diploma in Acupuncture and Anatomy (Sri Lanka)

- KPJAYI authorized ashtanga teacher (India)

- Certified intermediate series ashtanga Master Ji, Vishwanath Jois (India)

- Yoga Alliance EYRT 500 (USA)

- Yoga alliance YACEP (USA)

- Yoga Alliance RYS – Registered yoga school

- Founder Brahma Shakti Vinyasa Yoga

He and his wife Stephanie regularly conduct workshops, intensives and teacher training courses and are amongst China's favourite foreign yoga teachers. .

WHAT - ABOUT BRAHMA SHAKTI VINYASA YOGA

Brahma Shakti Vinyasa Yoga is a vinyasa flow practice, based on the 8 limbs of yoga and the traditional teachings of Krishnamacharya. It is tailored to suit the needs of the 21st century modern yoga practitioner, no injuries, no ego, no competition, just pure transformational yoga.

The Hatha Yoga Pradipika from the 15th century advises 'Vina vinyasa yogena asanadin na karayet' (translation 'Oh yogi, do not practice asana without vinyasa.')

Vinyasa encourages the practitioner to flow from one asana to the next in a rhythmical way following the breath. When this is linked with Bandha (body locks), we create internal fire burning the toxins we have accumulated in our daily lives, removing excess fat, adding tone to the body and making the skin shine. By using these four principles of Bandha, Drishti, Ujayi breath and Vinyasa we achieve meditation in movement and a truly life changing practice incorporating seven of the eight limbs of yoga.

Classes start with Japa mantra meditation to create a atmosphere of peacefulness and communal prana, continuing into vinyasa asana practice of sun salutation, standing series, sitting, back bending, inversions and ending in pranayama.

Many of the adjustments offered by the teacher incorporate myofascial and trigger point release techniques allowing the muscles to release and extend, removing blockages as blood flow is increased to the extremities of the body giving a therapeutic effect for general good health and well being.

WHY:

While living in Mysore for over 20 years and becoming dedicated to a life of yoga, initially through Hatha Iyengar style and then ashtanga at KPJAYI, I witnessed many ashtanga practitioners being granted the authority to teach without being given any formal education in adjustment or anatomy. All one had to show was a commitment to a regular yoga practice for a period of three to four years. The current scion of KPJAYI Sharath Rangaswamy (later Jois,) Sharath Yoga Centre. holds no knowledge of anatomy and only adjusts students in five asanas of the primary series, Utthita Hasta Padangusthasana, Ardha Baddha Padmottanasana, Marichasana, Supta Kurmasana, and Backbending. I have personally witnessed assistant teachers being screamed at for helping struggling students in any other than the permitted five asanas, I do not believe this is the correct way to teach and guide students in their progress.

In the present ashtanga system I have witnessed 'rigid' teachers overloaded with their own ego forcing students into uncomfortable positions or even injuring them. If someone could not complete a certain asana because of their body limitations they could get stuck at that asana for several years not being able to move forward into the following asana of the series. It was not always like this, both Pattabhi and Manju Jois allowed modifications and did not stop students from moving forward in the series, however due to the increased numbers of students visiting Mysore and the limitations of time, stopping students became the norm.

Vinyasa yoga practice dates back thousands of years and gives amazing benefits when approached in the correct way, respecting ones personal limitations.

In the modern yoga world where over 80% of practitioners are female I feel that modifications should be taught along with adjustments that respect personal boundaries.

I love the ashtanga system but as I grew older I needed a practice I could maintain, a 'sustainable practice' that still gave me the same benefits.

Yoga is in fashion at the moment but once started it should become a lifetime practice. That is our mission with Brahma Shakti Vinyasa Yoga, making practice enjoyable, where every student can evolve, applying the vinyasa system to meet the needs of everyday life, bringing about healthy, happy, humble Yogis spreading their positive energy, helping to make the world a better place.

I often found students joined my ashtanga workshops and trainings out of curiosity and they did not maintain a regular practice afterwards because they found it too demanding.

Students often raised the following questions and comments in class:

- "I am scared of ashtanga because it is too difficult"

- "Will a lady's body become like a mans and will I lose my breasts or menstrual cycle?"

- "I have heard Ashtanga yoga is only for young gymnastic people"

- "Will I get injured easily?"

I believe that a person get's injured at the hands of inexperienced teachers, and because their own ego creates a competitive environment. It does not have to be this way, at Brahma Shakti Vinyasa Yoga we aim to create professional teachers and practitioners so everyone can enjoy the benefits of vinyasa yoga in a safe environment for a lifetime.

SECTION 2: BANDHA, UJAYI BREATH, DHRISTI, VINYASA

THE BASICS OF BRAHMA SHAKTI VINYASA YOGA

BANDHA (BODY LOCKS)

The three bandhas used in Brahma Shakti vinyasa yoga are:

- Moola bandha – situated around the perineum/pelvic floor.

- Udiyana bandha – 2 inch or 3 fingers width below the naval.

- Jalandhara bandha – in the throat region.

MOOLA BANDHA: THE ROOT LOCK.

To find moola bandha:

- Sit on the floor in a padmasana or half lotus position.

- Feel the sitting bones touching the floor, draw them together towards the centre, then relax the buttocks without releasing the sitting bones.

- Now focus on the pubic and tail bone and bring them together into the same centre.

- Moola bandha is where these 4 points meet, draw the energy up from that point

To find moola bandha another way, imagine you are out and about and you suddenly feel the urge to go for a 'pee' - a number 1. You would consciously tighten the muscles in the pubic area, which would keep you from releasing.

Now imagine the same situation and you need to go for a 'poo' - a number 2. Again you would tighten the muscles, this time at the rear in the anal area to stop the release.

In between number 1 and number 2 is number 1½. This is the point where moola bandha is located. Now draw up the energy from that point, this is moola bandha.

First, we train the mind to recognize the muscle group, and then it becomes physical as the mind sends the message to the muscles and eventually it becomes automatic.

UDDIYANA BANDHA - ABDOMINAL LOCK

Uddiyana bandha is situated 2 inches, three finger widths below the naval.

To find uddiyana bandha:

Locate the place three finger widths below the navel. Draw in and hold, linking this spot with the top of moola bandha whilst maintaining inhalation and exhalation. With practice when you draw in udiyana bandha, moola bandha will automatically engage.

You should hold moola bandha and uddiyana bandha at all times, for example, whenever you are walking, driving or sitting, not just in your asana practice. When practiced consistently this will make your internal core strong, prevent urinary and intestine problems and protect the lower back, while maintaining good posture.

Do not confuse uddiyana bandha with Uddiyana bandha practiced in hatha yoga.

JALANDHARA BANDHA - CHIN LOCK

Jalandhara bandha is situated in the throat region; while as moola bandha and udiyana bandha seals the bottom of an imaginary tube, Jalandhara bandha seals the top.

To find jalandhara bandha

- Sit with moola bandha and udiyana bandha engaged, with a straight back and shoulders square.

- Lengthen your cervical spine then drop the chin towards the chest, not forcing. Do not just bend your chin and let your shoulders sink forward.

- By swallowing/ gulping once this completes the seal in the throat.

Jalandhar bandha is not engaged in all asanas as the other two bandhas are. It is used only in certain asanas.

UJAYI BREATH (BREATHING WITH SOUND)

Ujayi breath is simply breathing with sound (it is not the same as ujayi pranayama).

Stand tall or sit in half lotus position with a straight back, moola bandha and uddiyana bandha engaged.

- Close your eyes and exhale with the mouth open making the sound ahhhhhhh.

- Feel where the sound is coming from; you should feel a small vibration in the glottis (lower throat).

- Now repeat the same exercise with the mouth closed. The vibration and the internal sound is increased and more pronounced in the glottis, almost like a elongated sigh. Feel the length of the breath.

You should only hear the sound on the exhalation. It can be a soft noise that you alone can hear or stronger so that other people can also hear. Both are correct as long as you feel the vibration.

Try to create a rhythm with the breath and stay with it throughout the practice, like a mantra to focus awareness

The vinyasa series was created to burn the accumulated toxins from the body. With regular practice of vinyasa, bandha and ujayi breath you will create an internal fire burning up accumulated toxins in the body

All breathing should be done with the nose not the mouth.

DRISTHI (GAZING POINT)

Dristhi is the gazing point within the asana. It holds the attention, improves concentration and brings about a feeling of oneness, resulting in meditation in movement. There are different Dristhi used in different asanas.

Urdhva dristhi – up to space

Brumadhya dristhi – third eye (between the eyes towards forehead)

Nasarga dristhi - tip of the nose

Parsva dristhi - left side or right side

Nabhi dristhi - navel

Hastagra dristhi - tip of middle finger

Angusta dristhi - tip of the thumb

Padagra dristhi - tip of big toe

VINYASA

Vinyasa refers to the movements and breathing pattern within the sequence of the asana, one breath, one movement.

G. Mohan succinctly explains the modern meaning of vinyasa in his biography of his teacher T. Krishnamacharya (the teacher of BKS Iyenger, Desikacharya Pattabhi Jois and Indra Devi).

> "A special feature of the asana system of Krishnamacharya was vinyasa. Many yoga students today are no doubt familiar with this word – it is increasingly used now, often to describe the 'style' of a yoga class, as in 'hatha vinyasa' or 'vinyasa flow'. Vinyasa is essential, and probably unique, to Krishnamacharya's teachings. As far as I know, he was the first yoga master in the last century to introduce this idea. A vinyasa, in essence, consists of moving from one asana, or body position, to another, combining breathing with the movement."

SECTION 3: THE PRACTICE - JAPA MANTRA MEDITATION.

All classes in Brahma Shakti yoga start with Japa mantra meditation.

A Japa Mala contains 108 beads plus 1 large bead called a Meru. When you count the beads and complete one full cycle coming back to the Meru, you should never pass the Meru, rather start again in the opposite direction.

When doing japa with a mala we should not use the index finger as this is connected with the ego, the thumb and the middle finger should be used to count the beads.

> The thumb represents will power.
>
> The first finger represents ego.
>
> The second finger represents pride.
>
> The ring finger represents knowledge.
>
> The small finger represents humbleness.

Japa Mantra can be a separate practice from your asana practice. It is best done at a fixed time each day, dawn and dusk are the best times.

Sit on a mat in a comfortable position with legs crossed in a steady pose, back straight, eyes closed. Try to face northwards, by facing north in the direction of the mighty Himalayas spiritual currents will be mysteriously increased and benefit the practice by increasing the spiritual currents.

Do not do Japa in a hurried fashion; it is not the number of repetitions but the purity, concentration and mental attitude that help the practitioner attain the maximum benefit.

You can repeat the manta out loud or silently in your mind or just hum the melody.

Everything in the universe vibrates on specific wavelengths. The various mantras, although equally efficient, vibrate on different wavelengths. When we practice Japa we create a vibration ('prana', lifeforce or chi) that has a positive effect on ourself, the people around us, the space we are in and links us to the prana of the whole universe. The deeper the meditation the greater the prana.

In your own practice choose a favorite mantra that is personal to you. Sometimes your teacher will give you a mantra at the time of initiation. This is not saying one cannot recite any other mantras, sometimes the mind requires variety to counteract monotony, but your principal mantra should remain the same.

During meditation diseases of the mind such as lust, greed, hatred, anger, and jealousy are destroyed and replaced by pure thoughts. A beginner who is unaccustomed to the practice of mantra may find themselves giving up too soon after only a few minutes of repetition. However perseverance for around 30 minutes per day without interruption gives time for the mantra to work itself into the consciousness and the benefits will be felt within a few days.

By concentrating your internal attention on the third eye and picturing your favorite deity, Buddha, Ganesha, Jesus etc you can add tremendously to the effect. Sound and form reinforce each other but sound vibrations alone if practiced with clarity and devotion are capable of creating the same effect.

Repetition of mantra has a cumulative effect and with continued practice it gains more power.

It should be evident that Japa meditation is far more than just a verbal exercise; it is the state of complete absorption, and this energy can be a maintained at all times no matter what one is doing.

Various practical aids to progress in Japa meditation have been tried and tested for thousands of years and are based on psychological and natural principles handed down by ancient Seers.

Japa mantra meditation is the easiest way to enter meditation as the mind is focused on one point as in 'Dharana' single pointed concentration, the sixth limb of the eight limbs of yoga.

Japa mantra will help the mind steady itself, leading you towards true meditation and the state of oneness.

On a physical level many benefits are gained from Japa. Rest and relaxation are given to all the cells and organs of the body, toxins are removed and the nervous system is relaxed. The lower emotions are replaced by pure Sattvik thoughts.

Mantra meditation is an exact science like other forms of yoga. Sanskrit, the most ancient of human languages, is also known as Devanagiri, which when translated means 'language of the gods'. It is constructed of root sounds which are actual vibrations, in all languages the root sound 'Ma' or variations of this sound means mother which is usually the first word spoken by a child.

Sound made up of vibrations is energy, a Sanskrit mantra is a mystical, divine energy encased in sound. To release this energy we learn to repeat it at a certain rhythm, when we start repeating a mantra it creates a certain thought pattern in the mind that has a positive and calming effect.

There are different levels of sound, spoken and unspoken, the unspoken being the more powerful. The ancient seers, who were tuned into higher levels of consciousness were aware of the power contained in sound and the specific vibrations.

Mantras cannot be translated into other languages. Each mantra is constructed from a combination of sounds derived from the fifty letters of the Sanskrit language. No one sat down and wrote a mantra in the same way people write songs. Mantras are energy that always existed and cannot be created or destroyed. Discovered by ancient seers they have been handed down through the centuries.

This is similar to the teachings of Buddha, which were not learned by the Buddha himself but gained by divine revelation whilst in meditation beneath the Bodi tree at Bodhgaya in Bihar, India.

The science of mantra is an exact one and It is important that mantras are learned and pronounced correctly.

The sacred syllables used in mantra meditation are usually the Sanskrit names of the divine. Westerners are prone to think that certain mantras refer to different gods however these deities are all aspects of the one divine god, the ultimate supreme being in all religions, whose grandeur is too vast for the human mind to understand.

No practitioner, whatever their religion, contradicts their faith by practicing mantra. Mantra is merely a vehicle to attaining Samadi, enlightenment.

The root syllable 'man; in the word mantra comes from the first syllable of the word meaning to 'think' and 'tra' meaning to be free. Using them together they mean 'by thinking we free ourselves from the bondage of the world'. A mantra generates our creative force and brings eternal bliss. A mantra, when repeated constantly, awakens our deeper consciousness.

AUM is the original mantra. In Indian philosophical belief, God first created sound, then the universe arose from it. This first sound was AUM. The word AUM is three letters representing the three periods of time and the three states of consciousness.

> A is the waking state.
>
> U is the dreaming state,
>
> M is deep sleep.

When pronounced correctly 'A' is the first sound, starting from the naval with a harmonious vibration. As 'U' is pronounced the sound rises up to the mouth, 'M' the last sound rolls from the start of the tongue to the lips, closing the mouth.

AUM has a powerful positive effect upon the nervous system and transforms the physical body, awakening dormant physical and mental powers.

The universe came from the word AUM, rests in AUM and will end with AUM.

Aum can be used as a mantra itself but the mind must be very strong to be able to concentrate on a single world.

We use the following mantras in Brahma Shakti classes.

OPENING MANTRA

Om
Vande gurunam caranaravinde,
sandarsita svatma sukhava bodhe.
Nih sreyase jangalikayamane
samasara hala hala mohasantyai.
Abahu purusakaram sankhacakrasi dharinam.
Sahasra sirasam svetam pranamami patanjalim

Translation:
I bow to the lotus feet of the Gurus.
The awakening happiness of one's own self revealed,
Beyond better, acting like the jungle physician,
Pacifying delusion, the poison of samsara.
Taking the form of a man to the shoulders,
Holding a conch, a discus and a sword,
One thousand heads white,
To Patanjali, I salute.

Asatoma sadgamaya -
Tamasoma jyotir gamaya-
Mrutyorma samritan gamaya-
Om Shanti Shanthi Shanthi-

Translation:

From ignorance, lead me to truth

From darkness lead me to light

From death lead me to immortality,

Om, peace in me, peace in nature, peace in divinity.

Om Saha na vavatu -

Saha nau bhunaktu -

Saha viryam karavavahai-

Tejas vina va dhitamastu-

Ma vidvashavai

Om Shanthi Shanthi Shanthi.

Translation:

Om may we all be protected

May we all be nourished

May we all work together with great energy

May our intellect be sharpened

Let there be no animosity between us

Om. peace in me, peace in nature, peace in divinity.

Sri Rama Jaya Rama Jaya Jaya Rama

Translation:

Salutations to Rama, the great warrior and master of dharma

May my ego be purified, may my body be healthy and strong,
and may my past karmas be transcended.

Hare Kṛiṣhṇa hare Kṛiṣhṇa

Kṛiṣhṇa Kṛiṣhṇa hare hare

hare Rāma hare Rāma

Rāma Rāma hare hare

Translation:

Although the mantra is simply the recitation of three names,
its meaning has been translated as Oh Lord, oh energy of the Lord,
please engage me in your service.

Om shrim hrim klim glaum gam Ganapati eh namaha,
Sri Ganesh

Translation:

Let this world and all people of this world be good and have good.

Om gam Ganapati eh namaha

Translation:

Ganesha is known as the remover of obstacles, the mantra typically
translated as "salutations to the remover of obstacles.

Om
Bhur bhuvah svah
Tat savitur varenyam
Bhargo devasya dhimahi
Dhiyo yo nah prachodayat

Translation:

O thou existence Absolute, Creator of the three dimensions, we contemplate upon thy
divine light. May He stimulate our intellect and bestow upon us true knowledge.

Or more simply: O Divine mother, our hearts are filled with darkness. Please
make this darkness distant from us and promote illumination within us.

Shiva Shiva Shambho
Shiva Shiva Shambho
Maha Deva Shambho

Maha Deva Shambho.

Translation:

Glory to the Great Lord Shiva!
Thank Merciful! Glory to the one who brings
happiness and joy to live in the hearts of all!

Om Mani Padme Hum

According to Tibetan culture, it is said that
all the teachings of Buddha are contained in the mantra
Om Mani Padme Hum,
and that to know the mantra is to know Buddha himself.

CLOSING MANTRA.

Yogena chitasya, padena vacham
Malam sharirasya, cha vaidya kena
Yopakarotham, pravaram muninam
Patanjalim, pranjali ranatosmi
Ohm Brahma Shakti Namaha
Ohm Brahma Shakti Namaha
Ohm Brahma Shakti Namaha
Ohm

Translation:

I bow with folded hands to the supreme sage Patanjali, who eradicated the
impurity of mind with Yogashastra, impurity of speech with Vyakarana
Mahabhashya, and impurity of body with Ayurveda literature.

Bramha is the creator.

Shakti is devine energy.

To complete your mediation, sit silently for 3 to 4 minutes: clear the mind of all thoughts, find silence, internal focus at the third eye, hands remain in mudra resting on the knees, full yogic breath, straight back.

OBSTACLES TO MEDITATION

There are many obstacles to meditation, but you can overcome them with regular focused practice. The path of meditation is not easy, however the rewards far outweigh the effort and serve as a challenge to overcome obstacles.

Obstacles may include:

- Aimless wandering of the mind - keep the mind in check and bring it back to the source.

- Stopping practice - it is not always easy to adhere to a full practice but a little is better than none and keeps us on track to the final goal.

- Health - even if the body is ill, meditation can still be practised, influencing the mind towards regaining full health. "The mind is the best medicine"

- Diet - "we are what we eat" sattvik pure food is the best, processed food full of chemicals found on the shelves of the supermarket has no place in a yogic diet. Eating good pure foods locally produced in accordance with the seasons and eating moderately at the correct times is essential to advance in yoga and meditation.

- Laziness and sleep - when we first start to sit in meditation our muscles can easily become tired. This is easily overcome by regular practice of asana and meditation. Time spent in meditation is rewarded by the bodies requirement for less time spent in sleep. Twenty minutes meditation is equal to 1 hour of sleep; when we meditate regularly our body needs less time in sleep.

- Bad company, undesirable company - if we spend our time with negative people their energy may influence ours, the same way as television and movies with a violent theme influence us, these influences draw us to the negative not the positive.

- Useless conversation, gossip, bad talk - affect both our meditation and our karma.

- Self-justification - ego, I am.

- Anger, resentment, fury, irritation, attachment, lust and desire are enemies of peacefulness. - Often when we are in a state of anger we can say or do harmful things which cause a negative reaction. It is much better not to react. In the west we say "it takes two hands to clap". If we do not enter into argument no argument can occur.

- Doubt - when a student loses faith in the practice and its benefits, it is best to seek a experienced person who can guide them through this temporary obstacle.

SECTION 4: THE PRACTICE - ASANA.

PHYSIOLOGICAL BENEFITS OF ASANA

Our human body is the most advanced piece of machinery, correct maintenance keeps it going without problems through to old age.

Several 20th century yoga masters maintained health to their final years through the practice of yoga, they did not age prematurely and become old, they continued with their normal active life until it was time for them to leave the body.

Krishnamacharya 1888 to 1989 (101)

B K S Iyengar 1918 to 2014 (95)

K P Jois 1915 to 2009 (93)

Indra Devi 1899 to 2002 (102)

The practice of asana and pranayama is the way to preserve health and longevity of our body. Ashtanga yoga the eight limbs is unique in that it maintains the entire system and provides a soothing effect on both the external and internal body.

- Cells - no cellular exhaustion occurs, and the cells are made to free the body from toxins due to the internal massaging effect of asana. Blood flow is increased to the tissues and organs of the body, stopping the build up of free radicals.

- Mind - even modern medicine has now recognized the power of the mind over matter. The mind is kept in contact with the body during asana practice, making the practitioner's awareness more refined and able to identify any malfunction in any part of the body.

- Asanas work on both the gross and micro structures, skin, bone, muscle and connective tissue, etc. Asanas heal by their ability to increase circulation, open joints and tissue, and remove blockages and inflammation. As asanas contract and relax connective tissue and muscle, the strength and flexibility of both are increased.

- Due to the nature of movement in asana, the body is able to correct deformities in its structure by reshaping first the muscles, second the connective tissues, and finally the shape of the bones.

- Joints - asanas work on the joints by extending the range of movement and maintaining flexibility.

- Skin - the sensory nerve endings in the dermis are maintained due to the stretch given in asana, which in turn maintains the blood supply and tissue function of the epidermis, preventing premature aging. Yogis look younger than normal beings.

- Circulation is increased, allowing the blood to be delivered to all parts of the body.

- Cardiovascular and respiratory systems are kept healthy and efficient due to the massaging effect on the heart and lungs in asana. Blood supply and oxygen are processed at the optimum level, allowing healthy lymphatic flow, improving the supply of micro -nutrients

- Asanas massage the entire digestive system, promoting absorption and expulsion while maintaining healthy function of the pancreas, liver, kidneys and gall bladder.

- Yoga is the only system that has a beneficial effect on glandular function. Almost all the glands are massaged in asana, optimizing their function, endocrine, hypothalamus, pituitary, thyroid, ovaries etc.

- The nervous system reaches all parts of the body. In asana, the nerve roots are toned, maintaining healthy electrical transmission in the brain preventing senility. The Chakras relate to the autonomic nervous system that acts mainly unconsciously and regulates bodily function, such as heart rate, digestion, respiration, urination and sexual arousal, The Chakras, or energy centres, remain alert into old age, keeping the practitioner young, both in body and appearance.

- Ultimately, we can say yoga regulates all cellular functions of the body.

By practicing any form of vinyasa yoga 'movement combined with breath' while focusing on a single point we practice meditation in movement.

The combination of bandha and ujayi breath creates internal fire, which burns away the toxins we have accumulated in our daily lives.

Vinyasa is a traditional practice mentioned in the Hatha Yoga Pradipika, 'Vina vinyasa yogena asanadin na karayet (O yogi, do not do asana without vinyasa)'.'

Everyone can practice vinyasa yoga, maintaining optimum health if we respect our body and practice inside our limitations.

Yoga practice should never bring undue stress to the mind or to the body, respect your body and listen to signals sent by the nervous system, in this way you will continue your practice and enjoy the special time spent on you mat, while giving the maximum benefit to your body, mind and soul.

Pain and injury are not necessary parts of asana practice, ego is the creator of pain and injury, pushing you past your own personal safe limits.

"Leave your ego outside the practice room with your shoes".

ASANA POSTURE

In yoga, asana plays a very important role. Asana means posture, meant for successful meditation.

A stable and comfortable posture is the aim of Patanjali yoga in order to seek a merger with the universal soul. For the higher transcendent soul that rests in the body we need to develop the gross body. Patanjali recommends asana practice as a preparation for sitting in meditation.

These days, asana is often practiced only as a keep fit routine, which limits the students spiritual advancement. Posture enables the body to maintain health and helps to overcome obstacles associated with our daily modern lifestyle, but the greatest effects of asana are on the mind and soul.

Asana is a firm and comfortable posture, the yogi must be able to be in this posture without any discomfort or difficulty.

"Sthiram Sukham Asanam" (PYS 2.46)

Translation: Sthiram - stable posture, steady, motion-
less determined, well balanced and settled.

Sukham - highly invigorative, ease, causing no pain, provides comfortable breathing.

Asanam – asana, posure.

Sama Samastham - a single word to describe all the qualities of asana, it means, a balanced posture where no part of the body is under stress.

According to the Hatha Yoga Pradipika, the purpose of asana is to gain stability and wellness. By practicing yoga, anybody, young, old, or sick, will gain good health.

ASANA PRACTICE.

Asana involves 4 stages:

1. Doing stage of asana, moving into.
2. Being in asana.
3. Attaining total awareness.

4. Moving out of asana.

> 1 - The doing stage, moving into is preparation to reach the final stage of asana. You need to move, fold, flex our arms and our legs and bend our body in order to reach the final position.

Many students concentrate on the final position without thinking about the limitations of their body, thereby compromising the asana. It is better to reach as close to the final position as possible rather than to do the position incorrectly. The body needs time to reach the final position, enter correctly and advancement comes much quicker. Accept your limitations then you can progress in your practice.

> 2 - The being stage, in this stage you can stay in the final position (or as close as you can) for the assigned number of breaths, fix your dristhi and breathe with awareness. A stable and comfortable posture allows concentration.

> 3 - Stage of attainment, in this stage you get the highest awareness.

> 4 - Moving out of asana, often the mind is conditioned for the being stage, forgetting that coming out of the posture correctly without loss of focus is equally important.

AWARENESS IN PRACTICE

Awareness is the most essential, it can bring true knowledge and bliss by removing the ego. The ability to make the journey towards the higher self, connecting to the divinity around you is only possible through awareness.

The whole yoga process of the '8 Limbs' is designed to create total awareness. The building of awareness creates harmony in our system, allowing the body to be still (asana), to arrive at the breaths full potential (pranayama), and to maintain peace and presence of mind (meditation).

These qualities should be maintained in your daily yoga practice, by adopting the higher state of awareness while practicing, negative imprints on your karma accumulated throughout life are dissolved, by being in complete awareness no negative karmic imprints will be possible.

The stretch, balance, strength building, deep breath and focus cleans the blockages and is one of the best things that can happen in your life.

The yogi should learn to experience the subtle awareness which is very important in your yoga practice. You should learn to understand how your body works through these subtle changes using body awareness.

Comparing ourselves with others and trying to reach the same posture as others when our body is not ready, is due to 'ego' from our physiological conditioning. When your body is not ready it will revolt, resulting in injury. It is well known that the ego is separate from the physical body. When the ego is trying to influence the body, disharmony is created, that is why you feel pain and suffering, you are creating the 'cause' and also creating the 'effect' yourself.

When you are in the state of awareness and you do actions in the connected state, these actions flourish in harmony with the physical body, resulting in progress of your own personal practice, "It is not which asana you practice but how you practice asana".

It does not matter if you cannot do an asana as perfectly as someone else, we all have limitations. It is the state of 'being' in asana, in total awareness. Practicing in this way, will give the maximum benefits you should get from yoga.

OPENING MANTRA

Om

Vande gurunam caranaravinde, sandarsita svatma sukhava bodhe.

Nih sreyase jangalikayamane samasara hala hala mohasantyai.

Abahu purusakaram sankhacakrasi dharinam.

Sahasra sirasam svetam pranamami patanjalim

Translation:

I bow to the lotus feet of the Gurus.

The awakening happiness of one's own self revealed,

Beyond better, acting like the jungle physician,

Pacifying delusion, the poison of samsara.

Taking the form of a man to the shoulders,

Holding a conch, a discus and a sword,

One thousand heads white,

To Patanjali, I salute.

I have added one extra Suryanamaskar variation, which helps to strengthen and set the shoulders. This suryanamaskar is from the tradition of the Mysore Garadi wrestlers as practiced in the vyayamashalas. I have named it Hanuman Namaskar in respect to Lord Hanuman the God worshipped by the wrestlers for his strength and bravery.

HANUMAN NAMASKAR X 2

Samasthiti Position; Feet together, strong legs turn in the quadriceps, engage moola and udiyana bandha, open chest, hands by your side.

Step one

1. Inhale, raise the hands, stretching tall, turn in the triceps and lift from the elbows, dristhi thumbs.

2. Exhale, fold forward over the top of udiyana bandha, hands to floor.

3. Inhale, raise the head open chest.

4. Exhale, walk both legs back to chaturanga position, drop the knees. lower the shoulders.

5. Inhale, raise the shoulders and the hips back up, knees on the floor.

6. Exhale, take the hips back to balasana child pose.

7. Inhale, raise the hips, moving forward bringing the shoulders over the wrists.

8. Exhale, down, lowering the shoulders.

9. Inhale, raise the shoulders and the hips up, knees on the floor.

10. Exhale, take the hips back to balasana child pose.

Step two

11. Inhale, raise the hips moving forward bringing the shoulders over the wrists.

12. Exhale down, with awareness, lowering the shoulders, looking forward.

13. Inhale, raise the chest 'urdhva mukha', upward facing dog position.

14. Exhale back to balasana child pose.

15. Inhale, raise the hips, moving forward bringing the shoulders over the wrists.

16. Exhale, down, lowering the shoulders, looking forward.

17. Inhale, raise the chest urdhva mukha, upward facing dog position.

18. Exhale come to ardha mukha, downward facing dog position, take 6 breaths. Push down with the hands, raise the tailbone, pushback with the hips, lengthening the side trunk, udiyana bandha engaged, looking towards the naval, nabhi dristhi,

19. Inhale, walk forward feet to hands, head up.

20. Exhale, head down.

21. Inhale, stand up, raise the hands, stretching tall.

22. Exhale samasthiti.

Repeat full sequence one more time.

STEP ONE

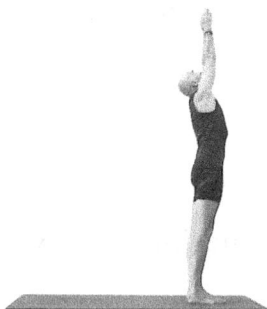

1. Inhale, raise the hands, stretching tall, turn in the triceps and lift from the elbows, dristhi thumbs.

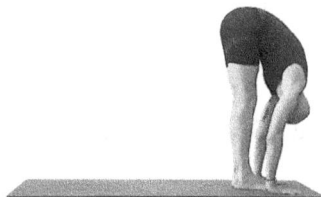

2. Exhale, fold forward over the top of udiyana bandha, hands to floor.

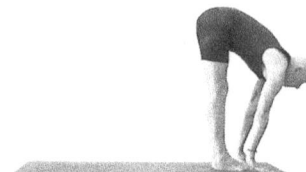

3. Inhale, raise the head open chest.

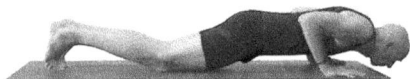

4. Exhale, walk both legs back to chaturanga position, drop the knees. lower the shoulders.

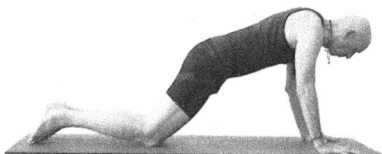

5. Inhale, raise the shoulders and the hips back up, knees on the floor.

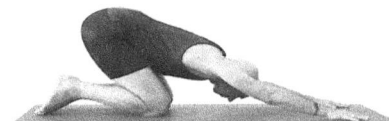

6. Exhale, take the hips back to balasana child pose.

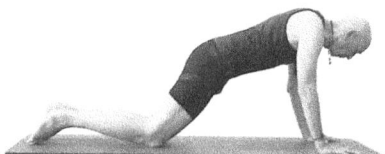

7. Inhale, raise the hips, moving forward bringing the shoulders over the wrists.

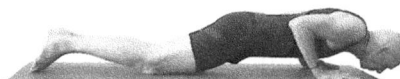

8. Exhale, down, lowering the shoulders.

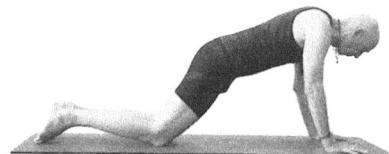

9. Inhale, raise the shoulders and the hips up, knees on the floor.

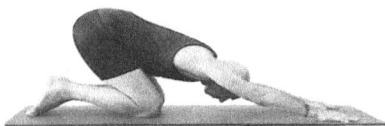

10. Exhale, take the hips back to balasana child pose.

STEP TWO

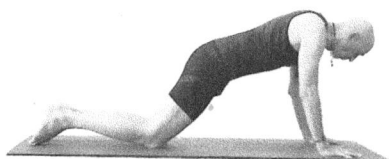

11. Inhale, raise the hips moving forward bringing the shoulders over the wrists.

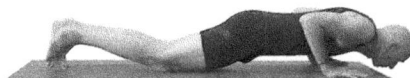

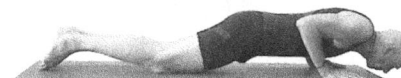

12. Exhale down, with awareness, lowering the shoulders, looking forward.

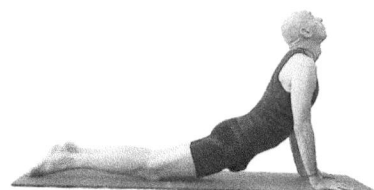

13. Inhale, raise the chest 'urdhva mukha', upward facing dog position.

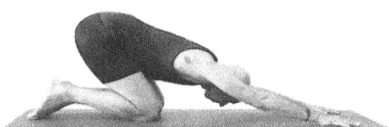

14. Exhale back to balasana child pose.

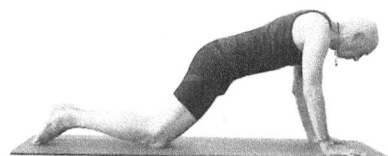

15. Inhale, raise the hips, moving forward bringing the shoulders over the wrists.

16. Exhale, down, lowering the shoulders, looking forward.

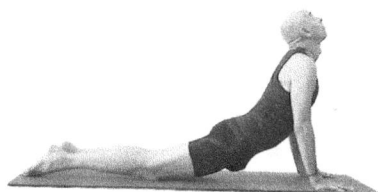

17. Inhale, raise the chest urdhva mukha, upward facing dog position.

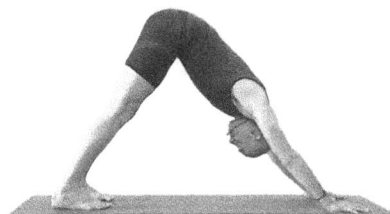

18. Exhale come to ardha mukha, downward facing dog position, take 6 breaths. Push down with the hands, raise the tailbone, pushback with the hips, lengthening the side trunk, udiyana bandha engaged, looking towards the naval, nabhi dristhi.

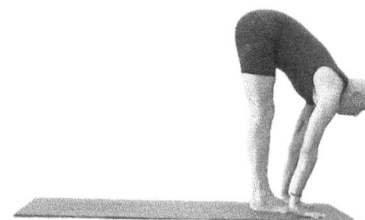

19. Inhale, walk forward feet to hands, head up.

STEP TWO (CONTINUED)

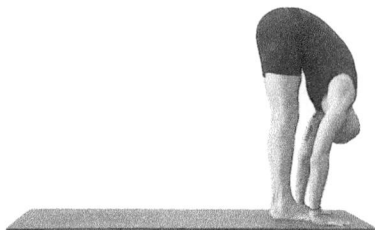

20. Exhale, head down.

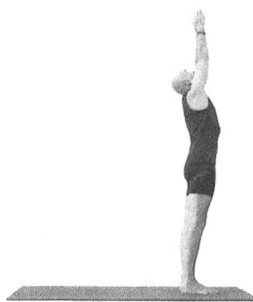

21. Inhale, stand up, raise the hands, stretching tall.

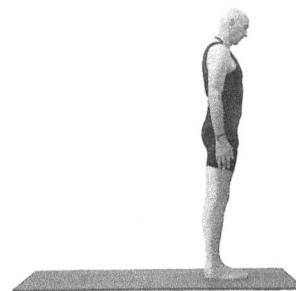

22. Exhale samasthiti.

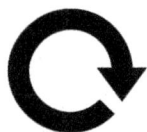

Repeat full sequence one more time.

SURYANAMASKAR A – SALUTE TO THE SUN. X4

Samasthiti Position; Feet together, strong legs turn in the quadriceps, engage moola and udiyana bandha, open chest.

1. Inhale – raise the arms and stretch tall lifting from the elbows extending the armpits and side trunk. This will allow the tissue to extend making jump through and binds easier later in the practice.

2. Exhale – fold forward from the hips, over the top of udiyana bandha locking udiyana bandha in place, extend the hands to the floor.

3. Inhale – head up only, strong legs

4. Exhale – jump or walk back into chaturanga, plank position.

5. Inhale – raise the chest, look up, urdhva mukha (upward facing dog), try to lift the thighs from the floor with feet flat and pointing back, push the pelvis down extending the lumber spine from the sacrum, lifting the thoracic spine (this is the first backbend) open the shoulders bringing the shoulder blades (scapula) down the back releasing the tension.

6. Exhale - raise the hips ardha mukha (downward facing dog), lift the tail bone, push back with the upper thighs, draw in uddiyana bandha, push down between the fingers and the thumbs, sending the energy up through to your hips, extending your side trunk, looking towards the naval, nabhi dristhi, take 6 breaths with sound.

7. Inhale - jump forward, head up.

8. Exhale - head down.

9. Inhale - stretch tall, raise both arms lifting from the elbows, looking towards the thumbs.

Samasthiti - Release, bring the hands down, stand tall.

Repeat the whole sequence Suryanamaskar A 3 more times.

Modifications:

2. Exhale, fold forward from the hips, catch the calves or ankles.

4. Exhale, walk back, lower the knees to the floor, bring shoulders over the hands, lower down to plank position, building strength in the shoulder girdle. Take an extra breath if required when going down. 2 chatwari knees down mod

7. Inhale walk forward to 2nd position, head up.

SURYANAMASKAR A

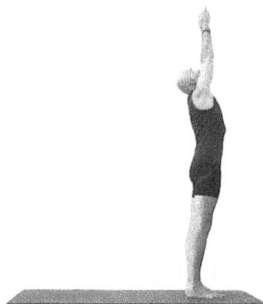

1. Inhale – raise the arms and stretch tall lifting from the elbows extending the armpits and side trunk. This will allow the tissue to extend making jump through and binds easier later in the practice.

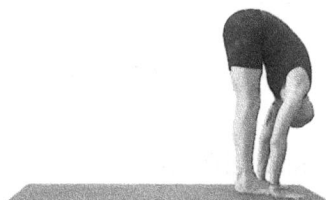

2. Exhale – fold forward from the hips, over the top of udiyana bandha locking udiyana bandha in place, extend the hands to the floor.

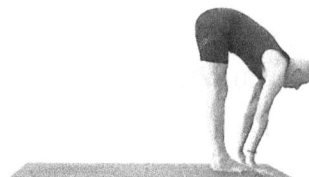

3. Inhale – head up only, strong legs

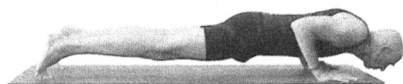

4. Exhale – jump or walk back into chaturanga, plank position.

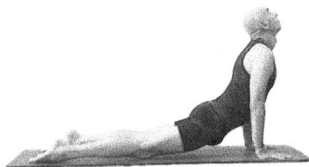

5. Inhale – raise the chest, look up, urdhva mukha (upward facing dog), try to lift the thighs from the floor with feet flat and pointing back, push the pelvis down extending the lumber spine from the sacrum, lifting the thoracic spine (this is the first backbend) open the shoulders bringing the

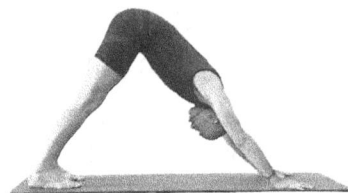

6. Exhale - raise the hips ardha mukha (downward facing dog), lift the tail bone, push back with the upper thighs, draw in uddiyana bandha, push down between the fingers and the thumbs, sending the energy up through to your hips, extending your side trunk, looking towards the naval, nabhi dristhi, take 6 breaths with sound.

SURYANAMASKAR A

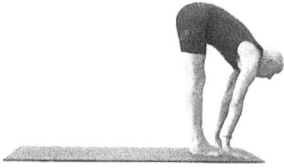

7. Inhale - jump forward, head up.

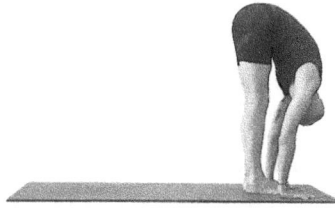

8. Exhale - head down.

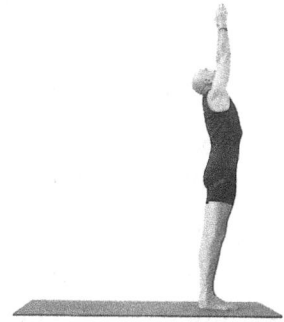

9. Inhale - stretch tall, raise both arms lifting from the elbows, looking towards the thumbs.

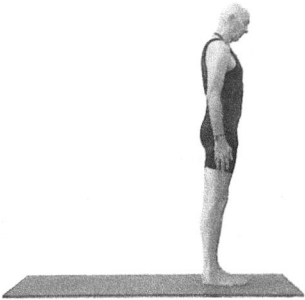

Samasthiti - Release, bring the hands down, stand tall.

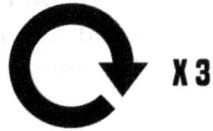

X 3

Repeat the whole sequence Suryanamaskar A 3 more times.

SURYANAMASKAR B X2

1. Inhale – bend the knees, stretch tall raising both arms lifting from the elbows looking towards the thumbs.

2. Exhale – fold forward from the hips, locking udiyana bandha in place, extend the hands to the floor.

3. Inhale – head up only.

4. Exhale – jump or walk back into chaturanga, plank position.

5. Inhale - raise the chest, Urdhva mukha (upward facing dog), try to lift the thighs from the floor with feet flat pointing back, push the pelvis down extending the lumbar spine from the sacrum while lifting the thoracic spine and sternum, open the shoulders bringing the scapula down the back releasing the tension.

6. Exhale – raise the hips, 'ardhva mukha' (downward facing dog).

7. Inhale – right foot forward, back foot at 45 degrees heel down, pushing the outside of the back foot into the ground, turning the thigh inwards engaging the quadricep. Right heel should be in line with the middle of the arch of left foot. Shoulders square, raise the arms lifting from the elbows, hands together, looking up towards the thumbs.

8. Exhale – all the way down into chaturanga, plank position.

9. Inhale - raise the chest, look up 'urdhva mukha' (upward facing dog), try to lift the thighs from the floor with feet flat pointing back, push the pelvis down extending the lower back from the sacrum, lifting the chest open the shoulders, bringing the scapula down the back releasing the tension.

10. Exhale – raise the hips , 'ardhva mukha' (downward facing dog).

11. Inhale - left foot forward, back foot 45 degrees heel down, pushing the outside of the back foot into the ground, turning the thigh inwards. Left heel should be in line with the middle of the arch of right foot. Shoulders square, raise the arms lifting from the elbows, hands together looking up towards the thumbs.

12. Exhale - all the way down into chaturanga, plank position

13. Inhale - raise the chest, look up 'urdhva mukha' (upward facing dog), try to lift the thighs from the floor with feet flat pointing back, push the pelvis down extending the lower back from the sacrum, lifting the chest, open the shoulders, bringing the scapula down the back releasing the tension.

14. Exhale - raise the hips ardha mukha (downward facing dog), lift the tail bone push back with the upper thighs, draw in udiyana bandha, looking towards the naval, nabhi dristhi, 6 breaths with sound.

15. Inhale – jump forward head up.

16. Exhale – head down.

17. Inhale – bend the knees, stretch tall, raise both arms lifting from the elbows, hands together, looking at the thumbs.

Samasthiti - Release, bring the hands down, stand tall.

Repeat the whole sequence Suryanamaskar B, one more time.

SURYANAMASKAR B

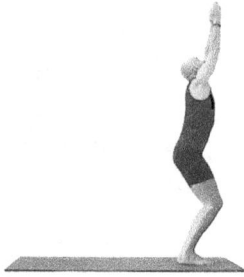

1. Inhale – bend the knees, stretch tall raising both arms lifting from the elbows looking towards the thumbs.

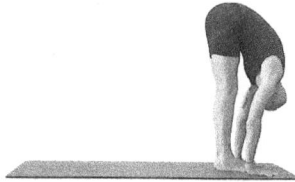

2. Exhale – fold forward from the hips, locking udiyana bandha in place, extend the hands to the floor.

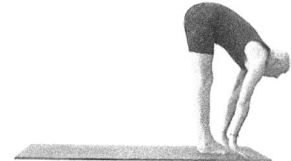

3. Inhale – head up only.

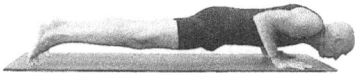

4. Exhale – jump or walk back into chaturanga, plank position.

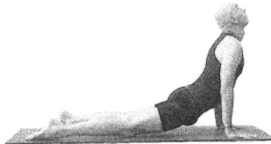

5. Inhale - raise the chest, Urdhva mukha (upward facing dog), try to lift the thighs from the floor with feet flat pointing back, push the pelvis down extending the lumbar spine from the sacrum while lifting the thoracic spine and sternum, open the shoulders bringing the scapula down the back releasing the tension.

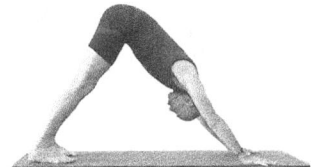

6. Exhale – raise the hips, 'ardhva mukha' (downward facing dog).

SURYANAMASKAR B

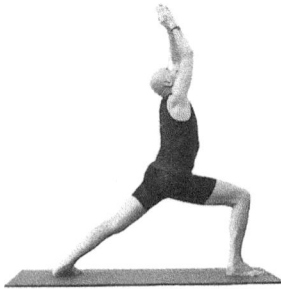

7.Inhale – right foot forward, back foot at 45 degrees heel down, pushing the outside of the back foot into the ground, turning the thigh inwards engaging the quadricep. Right heel should be in line with the middle of the arch of left foot. Shoulders square, raise the arms lifting from the elbows, hands together, looking up towards the thumbs.

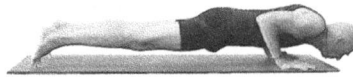

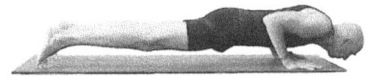

8. Exhale – all the way down into chaturanga, plank position.

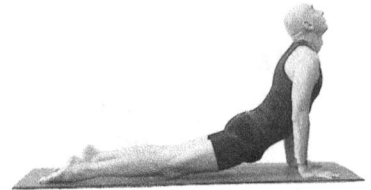

9. Inhale - raise the chest, look up 'urdhva mukha' (upward facing dog), try to lift the thighs from the floor with feet flat pointing back, push the pelvis down extending the lower back from the sacrum, lifting the chest open the shoulders, bringing the scapula down the back releasing the tension.

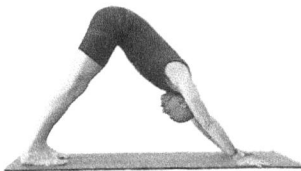

10. Exhale – raise the hips , 'ardhva mukha' (downward facing dog).

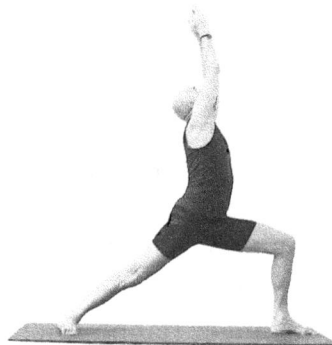

11. Inhale - left foot forward, back foot 45 degrees heel down, pushing the outside of the back foot into the ground, turning the thigh inwards. Left heel should be in line with the middle of the arch of right foot. Shoulders square, raise the arms lifting from the elbows, hands together looking up towards the

12. Exhale - all the way down into chaturanga, plank position

SURYANAMASKAR B

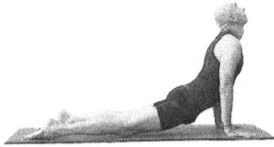

13. Inhale - raise the chest, look up 'urdhva mukha' (upward facing dog), try to lift the thighs from the floor with feet flat pointing back, push the pelvis down extending the lower back from the sacrum, lifting the chest, open the shoulders, bringing the scapula down the back releasing the tension.

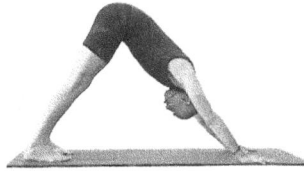

14. Exhale - raise the hips ardha mukha (downward facing dog), lift the tail bone push back with the upper thighs, draw in udiyana bandha, looking towards the naval, nabhi dristhi, 6 breaths with sound.

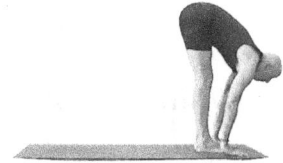

15. Inhale – jump forward head up.

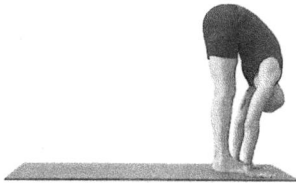

16. Exhale – head down.

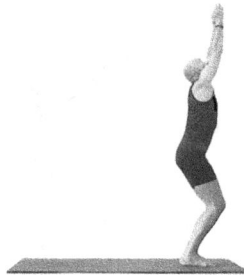

17. Inhale – bend the knees, stretch tall, raise both arms lifting from the elbows, hands together, looking at the thumbs.

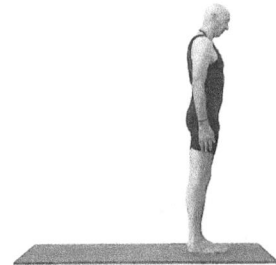

Samasthiti - Release, bring the hands down, stand tall.

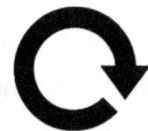

Repeat full sequence one more time.

Modifications:

4. Exhale - walk back, lower the knees, bring shoulders over the hands lower down, building strength in the shoulder girdle. Take an extra breath going down if required.

7. Inhale - right foot forward raise the arms, take an extra breath if required.

8. Exhale - drop the knees lower down with the shoulders. Take an extra breath if required. Repeat same technique left side.

STANDING SERIES OF ASANAS

PADANGUSTHASANA

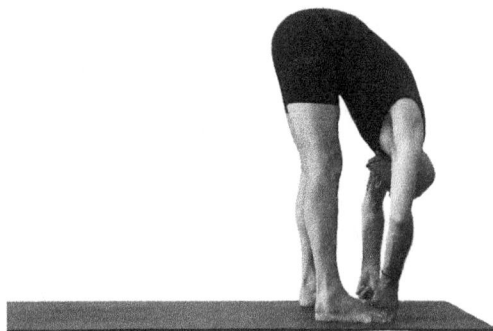

1. Jump the feet hip distance apart, hands on waist.

2. Inhale - catch the big toes, head up.

3. Exhale - fold forward, locking Udiyana bandha in place, crown of the head to the floor. Straight legs, turn in the quadriceps, raise the tailbone, bring the weight forward into the toes increasing the hamstring stretch. Open elbows out to the side, opening the chest. Take 6 or 9 breaths with sound. Dhristi nose.

4. Inhale- head up only, exhale

Modification:

If you can't catch your toes catch your calves or ankles and bend your knees slightly

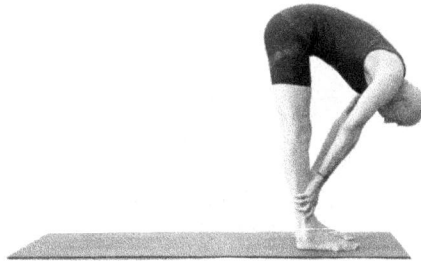

PADAHASTASANA

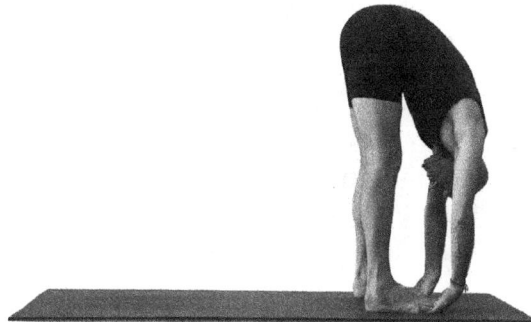

1. Inhale – place the hands under the feet, palms facing upwards.
2. Exhale - fold forward locking Udiyana bandha in place, crown of the head to the floor. Straight legs, turn in the quadriceps, raise the tailbone bring the weight forward more into the toes increasing the hamstring stretch. Open elbows out to the side opening the chest. Take 6 or 9 breaths with sound. Dhristi nose.
3. Inhale – head up only, exhale there.
4. Inhale - hands on waist come to standing position.
5. Exhale Samasthiti - jump the feet back together, release the hands   stand tall.

Modification:

> If you can't place the hands underneath the toes, catch your calves or ankles and bend your knees slightly

UTTHITA TRIKONASANA A

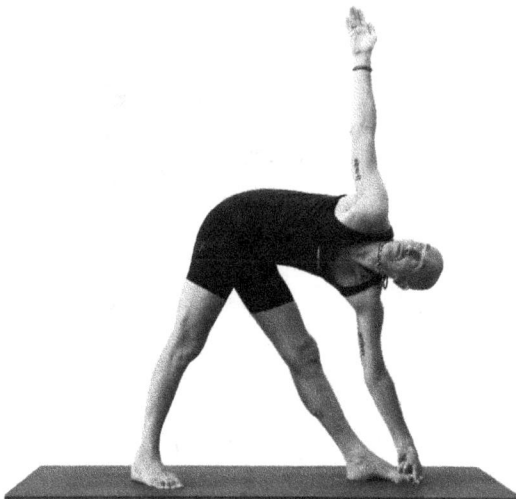

1. Inhale – jump or step the right foot to the right hand-side, arms out stretched, feet should be around 3 ft apart, or same length as your inner leg, right foot pointing forward back foot 45 degrees, right heel should be in line with the middle of the arch of the left foot.

2. Exhale – looking into the middle finger of the right hand, bend forward and catch the big toe of the right foot with 2 first fingers of the right hand, turn the right hip back, left hip forward slightly, engaging the legs. Raise the left arm and bring hand into dristhi line, open the chest, keeping the shoulders broad and the neck long. Take 6 breaths with sound. Dhristi left middle finger

3. Inhale – bring your gaze back to the right toe and come back to upright, arms outstretched turn feet back to parallel.

4. Exhale (photo) – turn left foot forward, back foot 45 degrees, left heel should be in line with the middle of the arch of the right foot, looking into the middle finger of the left hand, bend and catch the big toe of the left foot with the 2 first fingers of the left hand, turn the left hip back right hip forward slightly, engaging the legs. Raise the right arm and bring the hand in to dristhi line, open the chest, keeping the shoulders broad and the neck Long. Take 6 breaths with sound. Dhristi right middle finger.

5. Inhale – bring your gaze back to the left toe and come back to upright arms outstretched, turn feet back to parallel.

6. Continue into next asana.

Modification:

If you can't catch your toes, catch your ankles or calves

UTTHITA TRIKONASANA B

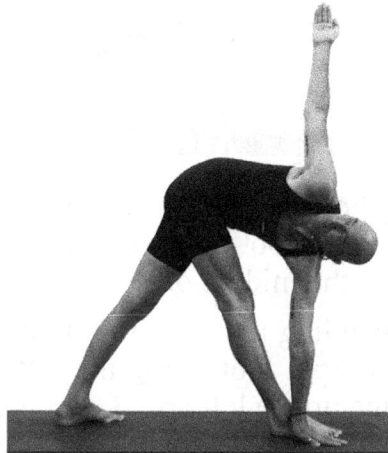

1. Exhale – turn right foot forward, back foot at 45 degrees, right heel should be in line with the middle of the arch of the left foot, bring the left hand over placing it to the right side of the right foot, raise the right hand upwards into dhristi line, opening the chest keeping the shoulders broad and the neck long. Take 6 breaths with sound. Dhristi right middle finger

2. Inhale – bring your gaze back to the right toe and come back to upright, arms outstretched, turn feet back to parallel.

3. Exhale – turn left foot forward back foot at 45 degrees, left heel should be in line with the middle of the arch of the right foot, bring the right hand over placing it to the left side of the left foot, raise the left hand upwards into dhristi line, opening the chest keeping the shoulders broad and the neck long. Take 6 breaths with sound. Dhristi left middle finger.

4. Inhale – bring your gaze back to the left toe and come back to upright, arms outstretched, turn feet back to parallel.

5. Exhale – jump or step back to front of the mat, lower the hands stand tall. Samasthiti

Modification:

If you can't catch your toes, catch your ankles or calves.

UTTHITA PARSVAKONASANA A

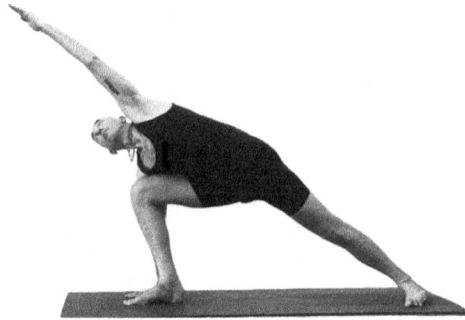

1. Inhale - jump or step to the right hand-side, arms out stretched, feet should be approximately 4 feet apart, right foot pointing forward, back foot at 45 degrees. Right heel should be in line with the middle of the arch of the left foot

2. Exhale - reach forward bending the knee to 90 degrees, lower the right hand to the floor on the outside of the right foot, bring the left hand over making a straight line from the left leg continuing up the left arm. Open the chest and torso, push down into the floor with the outside of the left foot. Make sure to keep the right thigh pointing straight forwards. Take 6 breaths with sound. Dhristi left middle finger.

3. Inhale - come back to upright arms out stretched, turn feet back to parallel.

4. Exhale - left foot pointing forward, back foot at 45 degrees. Left heel should be in line with the middle of the arch of the right foot. Reach forward bending the knee to 90 degrees, lower the left hand to the floor on the outside of the left foot, bring the right hand over making a straight line from the right leg continuing up the right arm. Push down into the floor with the outside of the right foot opening the chest and torso. Take 6 breaths with sound. Dhristi right finger.

5. Inhale - come back to upright arms out stretched, turn feet back to parallel.

Continue into the next asana.

Modification:

If you can't lower your hand to the floor let your elbow rest on your knee.

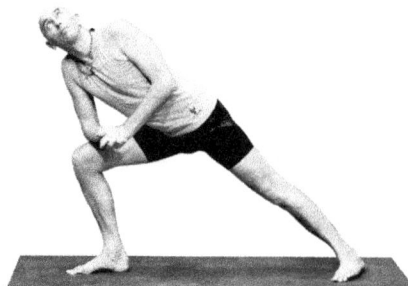

UTTTHITA PARSVAKONASANA B

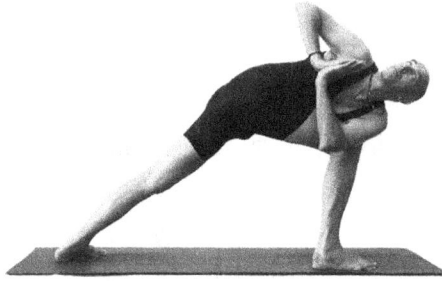

1. Exhale – turn to the right side, right foot pointing forward back foot at 45 degrees, right heel should be in line with the middle of the arch of the left foot, bend the right knee to 90 degrees, thigh pointing forward. Bring the left shoulder onto the right knee, hands together in prayer position, twisting the torso, open chest, Take 6 breaths with sound. Dhristi third eye.

2. Inhale - come back to upright arms out stretched, turn feet back to parallel.

3. Exhale - turn to the left side, left foot pointing forward back foot 45 degrees, left heel should be in line with the middle of the arch of the right foot, bend the left knee to 90 degrees, thigh pointing forward. Bring the right shoulder onto the left knee hands together in prayer position, twisting the torso, open chest. Take 6 breaths with sound. Dhristi third eye

4. Inhale - come back to upright arms out stretched, turn feet back to parallel.

5. Exhale - jump or step back to front of the mat, lower the hands, stand tall. Samasthiti.

PRASARITA PADOTTANASANA A

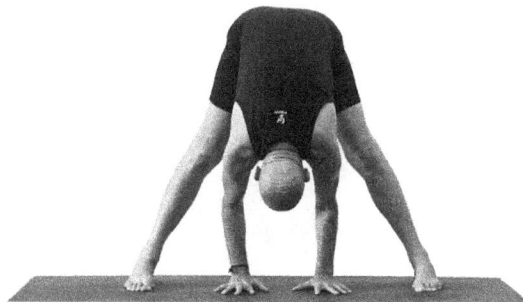

1. Inhale - jump or step to the right hand side, feet about 3ft apart, feet pointing straight forward or slightly inverted, hands on waist, lengthen spine, udiyana bandha engaged.

2. Exhale – fold forward, locking udiyana bandha in place drop the hands to the floor in line with your feet.

3. Inhale – raise your head, open chest, lift the tailbone, strong legs.

4. Exhale – fold forward finding space in your hips, straight legs, Take 6 breaths with sound. Dhristi tip of the nose.

5. Inhale – head up only, exhale there.

6. Inhale - come back up, straight legs, hands on waist. Exhale.

PRASARITA PADOTTANASANA B

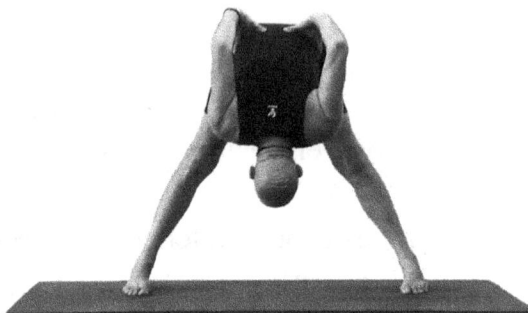

1. Inhale - arms out stretched.

2. Exhale - hands on waist,

3. Inhale raise the chest draw in udiyana bandha.

4. Exhale - fold forward over the top of udiyana bandha, finding space in your hips, straight legs, raise the tailbone, keep hands on waist, head towards the floor, take 6 breaths with sound. Dhristi tip of the nose.

5. Inhale - come back up, hands on waist, exhale there.

PRASARITA PADOTTANASANA C

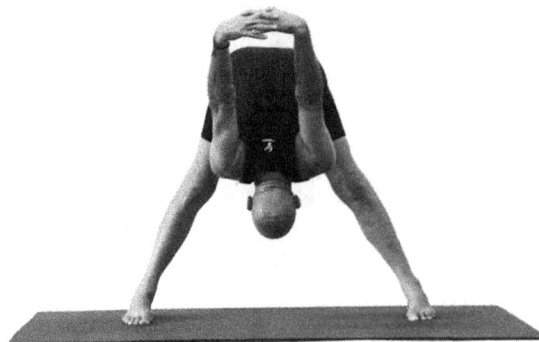

1. Inhale– arms outstretched.

2. Exhale – catch the hands behind the back.

3. Inhale raise the chest, draw in udiyana bandha.

4. Exhale - bend forward over the top of udiyana bandha crown of the head towards the floor, bring the arms towards the floor,behind the head, take 6 breaths with sound. Dhristi tip of the nose.

5. Inhale - come back up, hands on waist, exhale,

PRASARITA PADOTTANASANA D

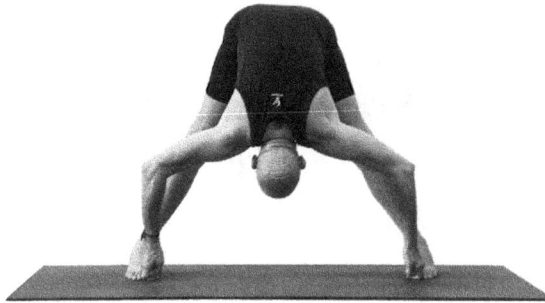

1. Inhale - hands on waist

2. Exhale – fold forward, catch the big toes with first two fingers.

3. Inhale raise the head, open chest, strong legs, lift the tailbone, draw in udiyana bandha.

4. Exhale - fold forward into the space you just created, crown of the head towards the floor, shoulders and arms parallel Take 6 breaths with sound. Dhristi tip of the nose.

5. Inhale - head up only, open chest, exhale there.

6. Inhale – come back up hands on waist.

7. Exhale - jump or step back to the front of the mat Samasthiti.

Modification for A, B, C, D:

If you can't lower your hands to the floor, put them on your calf and fold forward, lowering your hands down the legs as far as is comfortable.

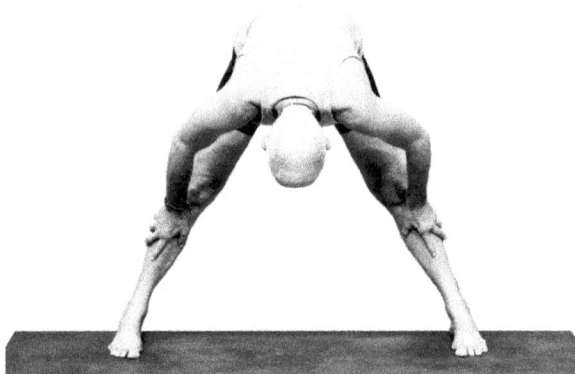

PARSVOTTANASANA

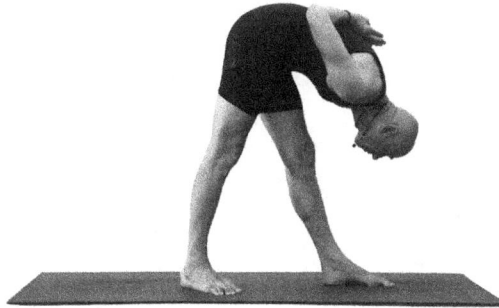

1. Inhale – jump or step to the right hand side, feet 2ft apart, Right foot pointing forward, left foot at 45 degrees, bring the hands together behind the back in reverse prayer position, square hips, square shoulders, raise the chest draw in udiyana bandha.

2. Exhale - fold forward, leading with the chest, chin to knee, engage the right big toe drawing the energy up into mula bandha, Take 6 breaths with sound. Dhristi right big toe.

3. Inhale – come back to upright, square hips, square shoulders.

4. Exhale - turn to the left hand side, left foot pointing forward, right foot at 45 degrees, fold forward, chin to knee, engage the left big toe drawing the energy up into mula bandha, Take 6 breaths with sound. Dhristi left big toe.

5. Inhale - come back to upright, square hips square shoulders.

6. Exhale – jump or step back to front of the mat release the hands. Samasthiti.

Modification:

If you can't bring your hands into reverse prayer, catch the elbows with hands.

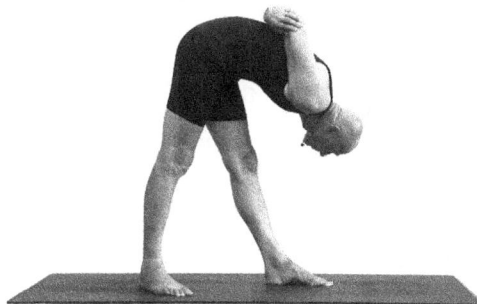

UTKATASANA

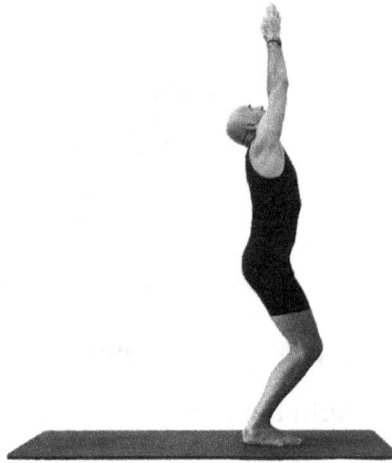

1. Inhale – raise the arms hands together, stretch tall lifting from the elbows extending the armpits and side trunk.

2. Exhale – fold forward from the hips, over the top of udiyana bandha, extending the hands to the floor.

3. Inhale – head up only.

4. Exhale – jump or walk back into chaturanga, plank position.

5. Inhale – raise the chest look up, urdhva mukha, (upward facing dog).

6. Exhale - raise the hips, ardha mukha, (downward facing dog).

7. Inhale – jump forward, bend the knees, raise both arms, turn in the triceps, lift from the elbows, hands together. Hands, shoulders, hips, ankles in a straight line. Take 9 breaths with sound. Dhristi thumbs.

8. Inhale – up, straighten the legs.

9. Exhale – fold forward from the hips, over the top of udiyana bandha, hands to floor, jump back to chaturanga, plank position.

10. Inhale – raise the chest look up, urdhva mukha, (upward facing dog).

11. Exhale – raise the hips, ardha mukha, downward facing dog.

Continue into next asana

VIRABHADRASANA A

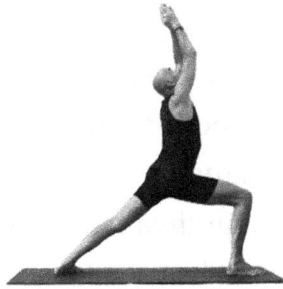

1. Inhale – bring right foot forward, turn left foot in to 45*. Bend the right leg, bringing the knee over the foot. Raise the hands above the head, turn in the triceps, lifting from the elbows to give maximum stretch, slight arch in the back, chest square. Take 6 breaths with sound. Dhristi thumbs

2. Inhale - straighten the right leg, turn to left hand side, left foot pointing forward, right foot at 45 degrees.

3. Exhale - bend the left leg, bringing the knee over the foot, Raise the hands above the head, turn in the triceps, lifting from the elbows to give maximum stretch, slight arch in the back, chest square. Take 6 breaths with sound. Dhristi thumbs.

Continue into next asana

Virabhadrasana A Modification:

Don't bend your knee too far, stay within your comfort zone.

VIRABHADRASANA B

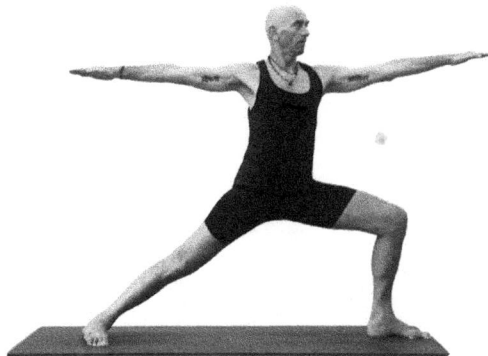

1. Inhale - open the arms parallel to the floor in line with the legs, do not come up, open chest, take 6 breaths with sound. Dhristi middle finger left hand

2. Inhale - straighten the left leg, turn to right hand side, right foot pointing forward left foot 45* keep the arms outstretched.

3. Exhale - bend the right leg, bringing the knee over the foot, arms outstretched, chest open. Take 6 breaths with sound. Dhristi middle finger right hand.

4. Inhale – take both hands to the floor on each side of the right foot,

5. Exhale - jump back lower to chaturanga, plank position.

6. Inhale – raise the chest look up, urdhva mukha, (upward facing dog).

7. Exhale - raise the hips, ardha mukha (downward facing dog).

Continue next asana.

Modification:

Don't bend the knee too far, stay within your comfort zone.

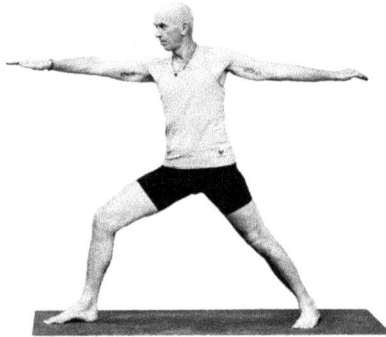

SITTING SERIES OF ASANAS

DANDASANA

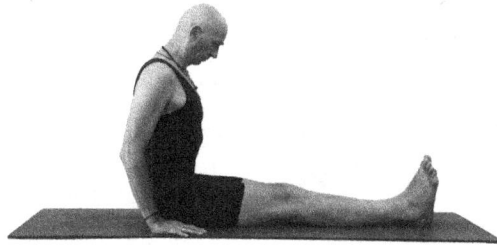

1. Sapta inhale – jump through to sitting position, straight legs, push forward with the heels roll in the quadriceps, moola and udiyana bandha engaged, straight back. Place the hands at the side of the waist pressing down with the palms, shoulders open. Lower the chin, engaging Jalandhara bandha, all 3 bandhas engaged. Take 9 breaths with sound. Dhristi nose.

PACHIMATANASANA A

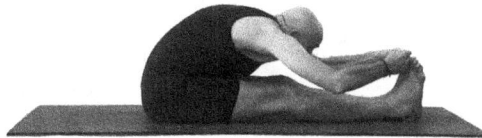

1. Inhale – catch the big toes with the first 2 fingers. Lengthen the spine, open the chest, head up.

2. Exhale – fold forward over uddiyana bandha, leading with the chest, chin to knee, maintaining length in the spine, open the elbows to the side opening the chest and shoulders, take 6 breaths with sound. Dhristi toes

3. Inhale – head up only, exhale there.

Modification:

Catch your calf or ankles, bend from the hips over udiyana bandha, extend the chest.

PACHIMATANASANA B

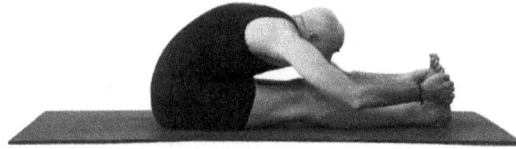

1. Inhale – catch the heels or bind catching the wrist with the hand, straight legs.
2. Exhale - fold forward over uddiyana bandha, chin to knee, maintaining length in the spine, open the elbows to the side, opening the chest and shoulders. Take 6 breaths with sound. Dhristi toes.
3. Inhale – head up only, exhale there.
4. Inhale - lift up vinyasa
5. Exhale - jump back to chaturanga, plank position.
6. Inhale - lift the chest urdhva mukha (upward facing dog).
7. Exhale - raise the hips, ardha mukha (downward facing dog).

Modification:

>   Catch your calf or ankles, bend from your hips over udiyana bandha, extend your chest, open the elbows.

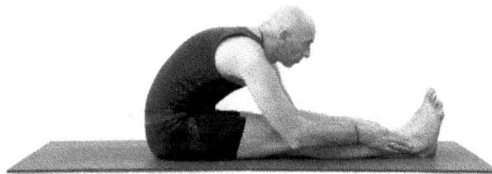

ARDHA BADHA PADMA PACHIMATANASANA – HALF BOUND LOTUS FORWARD BEND

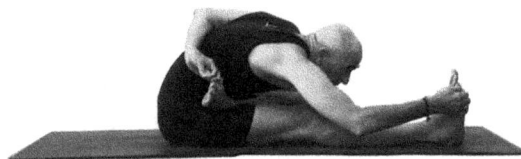

1. Inhale – jump through to sitting take the right leg into half lotus position, bring the right arm round the back and catch the right foot, square shoulders, maintain length in the torso, udiyana bandha engaged.
2. Exhale – fold forward leading with the chest, chin to knee, straight spine, catch left

foot with the left hand, open elbow, do not rest the arm on the floor. 6 breaths with sound. Dhristi left big toe.

3. Inhale – head up only, exhale there.

4. Inhale – Change to left side, take the left leg into half lotus position, bring the left arm round the back and catch the left foot, square shoulders, maintain length in the torso, udiyana bandha engaged.

5. Exhale - fold forward Take 6 breaths with sound. Dhristi right big toe.

6. Inhale - head up only, exhale there.

7. Inhale - lift up vinyasa

8. Exhale - jump back to chaturanga, plank position

9. Inhale - lift the chest urdhva mukha (upward facing dog).

10. Exhale - raise the hips ardha mukha (downward facing dog).

Modifications:

Bring your right leg in to half lotus, fold forward with both hands to try catch the foot.

If you can't catch your right foot with your right hand use a towel to help catch, fold forward.

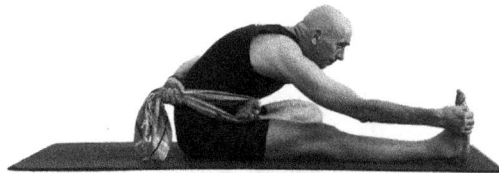

TIRYANGMUKHA EKAPADA PACHIMATANASANA – THREE LIMBED FORWARD POSE

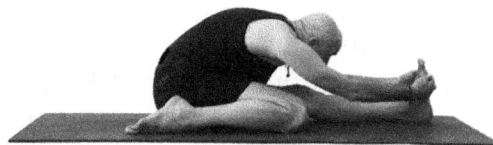

1. Inhale - jump through to sitting, take the right leg back, top of the foot on the floor, foot pointing backwards, square shoulders maintain length in the torso.

2. Exhale – fold forward chin to knee, leading with the chest, straight spine, catch the left foot with both hands or bind catching the left wrist with the right hand, resist

the urge to lean over to the left side leading with the left shoulder, open the elbows to allow a deeper fold, do not rest the arms on the floor. Take 6 breaths with sound. Dhristi left big toe.

3. Inhale – head up only, exhale there.

4. Inhale – change to left side, take the left leg back, square shoulders maintain length in the torso.

5. Exhale - fold forward chin to knee, leading with the chest, straight spine, catch the right foot with both hands or bind catching the right wrist with the left hand. Take 6 breaths with sound. Dhristi left big toe.

6. Inhale - head up only, exhale there.

7. Inhale - lift up vinyasa

8. Exhale - jump back to chaturanga, plank position.

9. Inhale - lift the chest, urdhva mukha (upward facing dog).

10. Exhale - raise the hips, ardha mukha (downward facing dog).

Modifications:

Fold your towel and place it under the sitting bone of the straight leg.

If you can't catch your feet, catch your ankle or calf.

JANUSIRSASANA A – HEAD TO KNEE POSE.

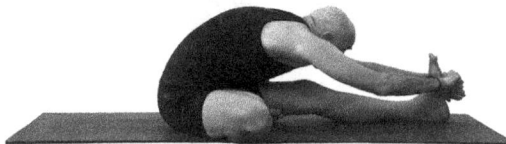

A, B and C can be combined with only vinyasa at the start and the end of the Janusirsasana series as was originally taught in Mysore.

1. Inhale - jump through to sitting, bring the right heel to the inside of the left leg, heel towards the anus, knee open out to the right side, square hips, square shoulders maintain length in the torso, udiyana bandha engaged.

2. Exhale – fold forward chin to shin, leading with the chest, straight spine, catch the left foot with both hands or bind catching the left wrist with the right hand, as you fold forward the right heel should put pressure on the perineum. Open the elbows to allow a deeper fold, do not rest the arms on the floor. Take 6 breaths with sound. Dhristi left big toe.

3. Inhale – head up only, exhale there.

4. Inhale – change to left side, bring the left heel to the inside of the right leg, heel towards the anus, knee open out to the right side, square hips, square shoulders.

5. Exhale – fold forward chin to shin, leading with the chest, straight spine, catch the right foot with the both hands or bind, as you fold forward the right heel should put pressure on the perineum. Open the elbows to allow a deeper fold. Take 6 breaths with sound. Dhristi right big toe.

6. Inhale - head up only, exhale there.

7. Inhale – enter next asana.

Modification

If you can't catch the feet, catch your ankles or calf muscles or use a towel to intensify the stretch.

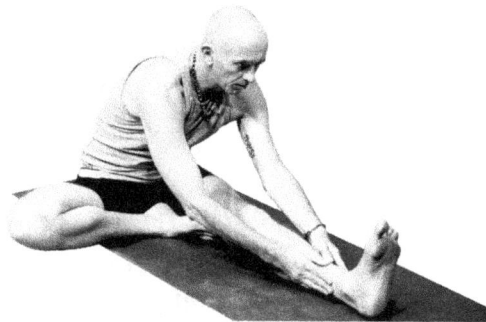

JANUSIRSASANA B

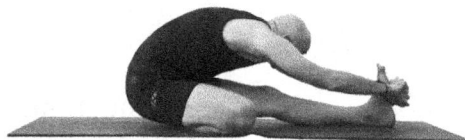

1. Inhale - bring the right foot up as in A, but this time the heel goes behind the anus, foot pointing forward, knee open out to the right side, square hips, square shoulders maintain length in the torso, engage udiyana bandha.

2. Exhale – fold forward chin to knee, leading with the chest, straight spine, catch the left foot with the hands or bind catching the left wrist with the right hand, open the elbows to allow a deeper fold, do not rest the arms on the floor. Take 6 breaths with sound. Dhristi left toe.

3. Inhale – head up only, exhale there.

4. Inhale – change to left side, bring the left heel behind the anus, foot pointing forward, knee open out to the left side, square hips.

5. Exhale - fold forward leading with the chest, straight spine, catch the right foot with both hands or bind, chin to knee Take 6 breaths with sound. Dhristi toe.

6. Inhale – head up only, exhale there.

7. Inhale – enter next asana.

Modification

If you can't catch the feet, catch your ankles or calf muscles or use a towel to intensify the stretch.

JANUSIRSASANA C

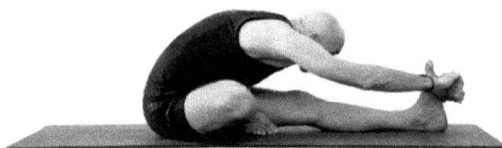

1. Inhale - bring the right heel onto the left thigh, twist the ankle, toes to the floor, push down with big toe, knee open out to the right side, square hips, square shoulders maintain length in the torso, udiyana bandha engaged.

2. Exhale – fold forward chin to knee, leading with the chest, straight spine, catch the left foot with the both hands or bind catching the left wrist with the right hand, open the elbows to allow a deeper fold, do not rest the arms on the floor. Take 6 breaths with sound. Dhristi left toe.

3. Inhale – head up only, exhale there.

4. Inhale – change to left side, bring the left heel onto the right thigh, twist the ankle, toes to the floor, knee open out to the left side, square hips, square shoulders maintain length in the torso.

5. Exhale – fold forward leading with the chest, straight spine, catch the right foot with the both hands or bind, Open the elbows to allow a deeper fold. Take 6 breaths with sound. Dhristi right toe.

6. Inhale – head up only, exhale there.

7. inhale - lift up vinyasa.

8. Exhale - jump back to chaturanga, plank position.

9. Inhale - lift the chest, urdhva mukha (upward facing dog).

10. Exhale - raise the hips, ardha mukha (downward facing dog).

Modification

First get used to the ankle and toes bending into position, don't fold forward, feel the stretch in the foot, take 6 breaths there. Slowly increase flexibility by bending forward a little more each day.

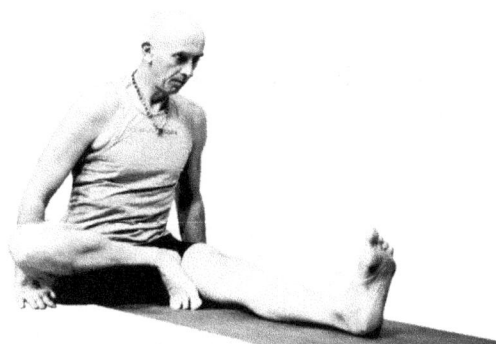

PARIGHASANA

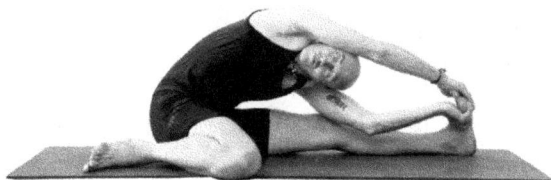

1. Inhale - jump through to sitting, take the right leg back with the foot behind the right hip. Left leg straight, place the hands on the floor between the thighs.

2. Exhale – lower the left shoulder towards the inner left knee, open the chest, take the right hand and catch the outside of the left foot, take the left hand and catch the palm to the arch of the foot, take 6 breaths, dhristi to the sky. Do not rest shoulder on the leg or arms on the floor.

3. Inhale – release the twist, keeping hold of the foot, look forward, exhale there.

4. Inhale, release, change to left side, take the left leg back with the foot behind the left hip. right leg straight, place the hands on the floor between the thighs.

5. Exhale – lower the right shoulder towards the inner right knee, open the chest, take the left hand and catch the outside of the right foot, take the right hand and catch the palm to the arch of the foot, take 6 breaths, dhristi to the sky. Do not rest shoulder on leg or arms on the floor.

6. Inhale – release the twist, keeping hold of the foot, look forward, exhale there.

7. Inhale – up vinyasa

8. Exhale - jump back to chaturanga, plank position.

9. Inhale - lift the chest, urdha mukha (upward facing dog).

10. Exhale - raise the hips, ardha mukha (downward facing dog).

MARICHASANA A – POSE DEDICATED TO SAGE MARICHI

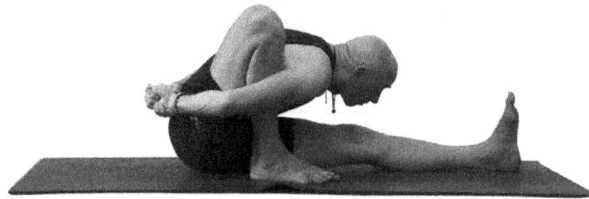

The marichasana series can also be grouped together with vinyasa only entering and exiting the series.

1. Inhale - jump through to sitting, raise the right knee, leave space between the foot and the thigh. Raise the right arm lengthening the torso, stretch forward taking the right arm round the right leg, bring the left arm round the back catching the right hand, sitting bones on the floor.

2. Exhale - fold forward chin to knee, leading with the chest, straight spine. Resist the urge to lift the sitting bone, draw in udiyana bandha and extend forward, take 6 breaths with sound. Dhristi big toe of left foot.

3. Inhale – head up only, exhale there.

4. Inhale – change to left side, raise the left knee, leave space between the foot and the thigh. Raise the left arm lengthening the torso, stretch forward taking the left arm round the left leg, bring the right arm round the back catching the left hand, sitting bones down.

5. Exhale - fold forward chin to knee, leading with the chest, do not raise the sitting bones, straight spine. Take 6 breaths with sound. Dhristi big toe of right foot,

6. Inhale – head up only, exhale there.

7. Inhale – enter next asana

Modification

If you can't catch the hands together, use a towel.

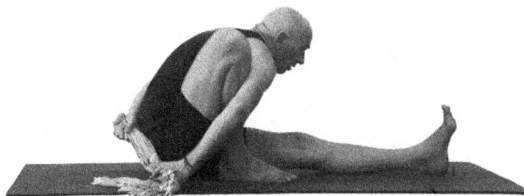

MARICHASANA B

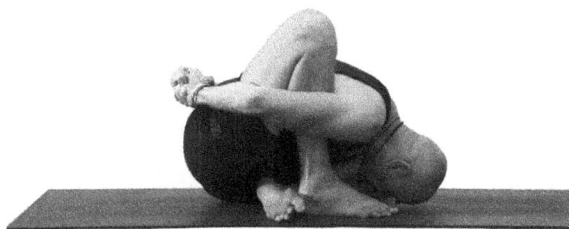

1. Inhale - raise the right knee bringing the left foot under the right knee, raise the right arm lengthening the torso, stretch forward taking the right arm round the right leg, bring the left arm round the back catching the right hand.

2. Exhale - fold forward, forehead to the floor. Take 6 breaths with sound. Dhristi tip of the nose.

3. Inhale – head up only, exhale there.

4. Inhale – change left side, raise the left knee bringing the right foot under the left knee, raise the left arm lengthening the torso, stretch forward taking the left arm round the left leg, bring the right arm round the back catching the left hand.

5. Exhale - fold forward, forehead to the floor. Take 6 breaths with sound. Dhristi tip of the nose.

6. Inhale – head up only, exhale there.

7. Inhale – enter next asana

Modification

If you can't catch the hands together, use a towel.

MARICHASANA C

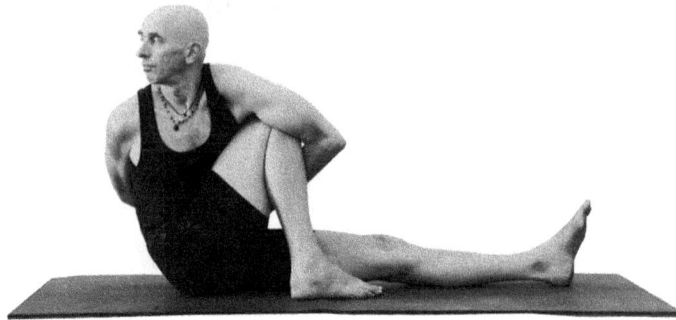

1. Inhale - raise the right knee, leave space between the foot and the thigh. Raise the left hand lengthening the torso, twist from the waist, take the left arm round the outside of the right leg, bend the elbow taking the arm back, bring the right arm round the back catching the left hand. Open the chest and shoulders lengthening the side trunk, look over the right shoulder. Take 6 breaths with sound. Dhristi into the distance.

2. Exhale - release

3. Inhale – change to left side, raise the left knee, leave space between the foot and the thigh. Raise the right hand lengthening the torso, twist from the waist, take the right arm round the outside of the left leg, bend the elbow taking the arm back, bring the left arm round the back catching the right hand. Open the chest and shoulders lengthening the side trunk, look over the left shoulder. Take 6 breaths with sound. Dhristi into the distance

4. Exhale - release,

5. Inhale – enter next asana.

Modifications:

If you have trouble bending the elbow and catching, leave the right hand on the floor, with left arm outside the right knee.

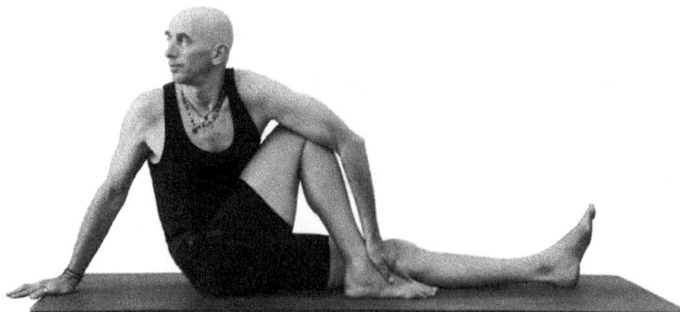

MARICHASANA D

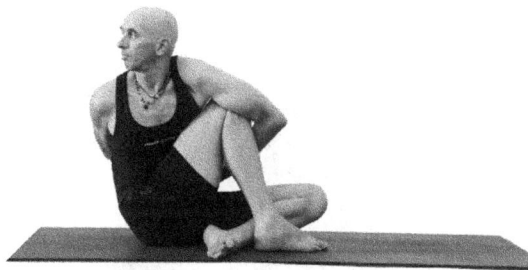

1. Inhale - raise the right knee bringing the left foot under the right knee, raise the left hand lengthening the torso, twist from the waist, take the left arm round the outside of the right leg, bend the elbow taking the arm back, bring the right arm round the back catching the left hand. Open the chest and shoulders lengthening the side trunk, look over the right shoulder. Take 6 breaths with sound. Dhristi into the distance.

2. Exhale - release

3. Inhale – change to left side, raise the left knee bringing the right foot under the left knee, raise the right hand lengthening the torso, twist from the waist, take the right arm round the outside of the left leg, bend the elbow taking the arm back, bring the left arm round the back catching the right hand. Open the chest and shoulders lengthening the side trunk, look over the left shoulder. Take 6 breaths with sound. Dhristi into the distance.

4. Exhale - release

5. Inhale - up vinyasa.

6. Exhale - jump back to chaturanga, plank position.

7. Inhale - lift the chest, urdha mukha (upward facing dog).

8. Exhale - raise the hips, ardha mukha (downward facing dog).

Modification

Bring the left leg under the right knee, raise the right knee, take the right arm back, with left arm outside the right knee, take 6 breaths.

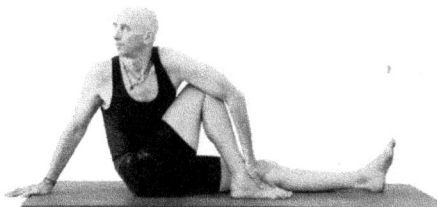

ARDHA MATSYENDRASANA

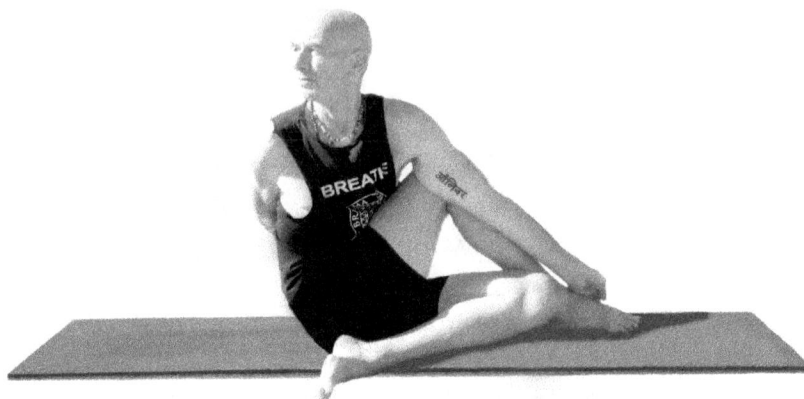

1. Inhale - jump through to sitting, raise the right knee bringing the left knee under the right knee, right foot on the outside of the left knee, raise the left hand lengthening the torso, twist from the waist, take the left arm down and catch the inside of the right foot, bring the right arm round the back, hand on to left thigh. Open the chest and shoulders lengthening the side trunk, look over the right shoulder. Take 6 breaths with sound. Dhristi into the distance.

2. Exhale - release

3. Inhale - change to left side, raise the left knee bringing the right foot under the left knee, raise the right hand lengthening the torso, twist from the waist, take the right arm down and catch the inside of the left foot, bring the left arm round the back, hand on to right thigh. Open the chest and shoulders lengthening the side trunk, look over the right shoulder. Take 6 breaths with sound. Dhristi into the distance.

4. Exhale - release

5. Inhale - up vinyasa.

6. Exhale - jump back to chaturanga, plank position.

7. Inhale - lift the chest, urdha mukha (upward facing dog).

8. Exhale - raise the hips, ardha mukha (downward facing dog).

Modification

Catch the right ankle with the left hand, take the right hand behind the back opening the chest, straight spine.

GOMUKHASANA – COW FACE POSTURE.

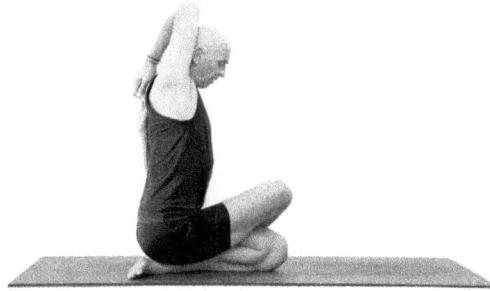

1. Inhale – Jump through to sitting, bring the left heel under the anus, sit on the left heel, bring the right knee over the left knee, fold the left arm up the back, raise the right arm, fold at the elbow and catch the hands together, lengthen spine, all 3 bandhas engaged, take 9 breaths. Dhristi tip of the nose.

2. Exhale – release.

3. Inhale - change to left side, bring the right heel under the anus, sit on the right heel, bring the left knee over the right knee, fold the right arm up the back, raise the left arm, fold at the elbow and catch the hands together, lengthen spine, all 3 bandhas engaged, take 9 breaths, Dhristi tip of the nose

4. Exhale- release

5. Inhale – up vinyasa

6. Exhale - jump back in to chaturanga, plank position.

7. Inhale - lift the chest, urdha mukha (upward facing dog).

8. Exhale -raise the hips, ardha mukha (downward facing dog).

Modification

Use a strap or towel if you can not catch the hands together yet.

NAVASANA – BOAT POSE 9 BREATHS X 3

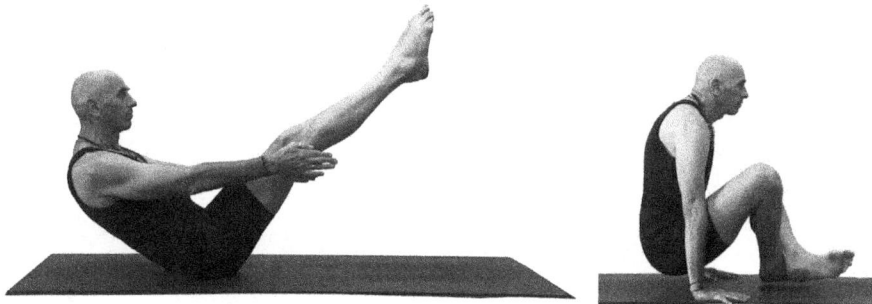

1. Inhale - jump through, raise the legs feet pointing forward just above eye level, arms straight and parallel to the floor, palms facing each other, lift the chest, udiyana bandha engaged, Take 9 breaths with sound. Dhristi, tip of the big toe. Exhale down.

2. Inhale - lift the buttocks from the floor with crossed legs, exhale down.

3. Inhale - again up to navasana position 9 breaths, repeat 1 more time, 3 times total.

4. Exhale - jump back to chaturanga, plank position.

5. Inhale - lift the chest, urdha mukha (upward facing dog).

6. Exhale -raise the hips, ardha mukha (downward facing dog).

Modification

If you are feeling too much strain with straight legs, bend the knees slightly, while keeping the arms outstretched,

If you get too tired catch the hands on legs.

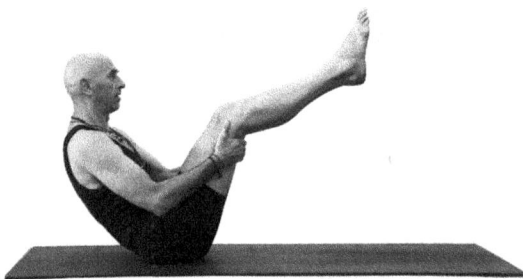

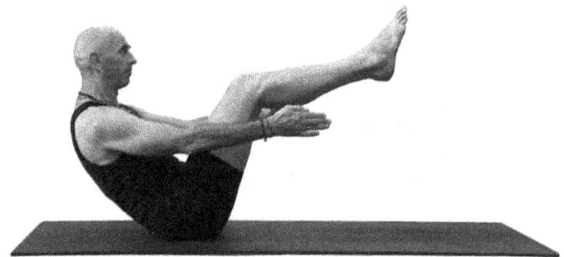

BADDHA KONASANA A – BOUND ANGLE POSE

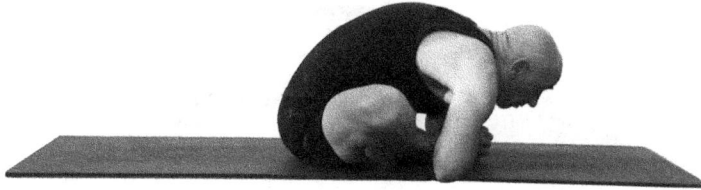

Baddha konasana, upavistha and supta konasana can be linked as a set with vinyasa only after completing all three.

1. Inhale - jump through to sitting position, bring the feet together up towards groin, knees out to side, spread the balls of the feet with the thumbs, raise the chest, engage udiyana bandha.
2. Exhale - bend forward, straight back, chin to floor, leading with the chest. Take 9 breaths with sound. Dhristi tip of the nose.
3. Inhale - come back to upright.

Continue to next asana.

BADDHA KONASANA B

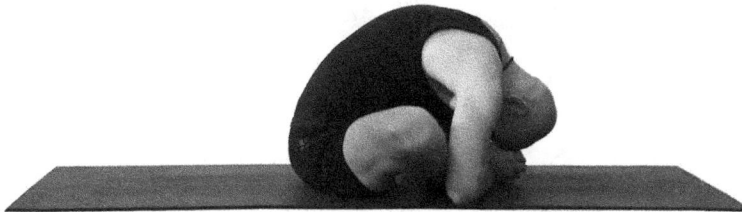

1. Exhale - touch the head to the toes arching the back, keep the balls of the feet open with the thumbs. Take 9 breaths with sound. Dhristi tip of the nose.
2. Inhale - come back to upright, exhale.
3. Inhale – enter next asana

Modification

Only bend forward to your own limit in both variations.

UPAVISTHA KONASANA A – WIDE ANGLE SEATED FORWARD BEND

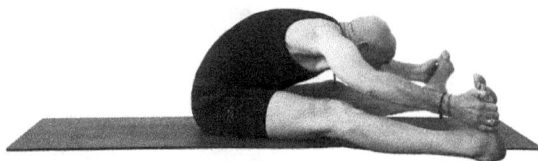

1. Inhale - spread the legs, catch the outside of the feet with the hands, head up.

2. Exhale - fold forward chin to floor, leading with the chest, take 6 breaths with sound. Dhristi tip of the nose.

3. Inhale - head up only, exhale there.

Continue into Upavistha konasana B

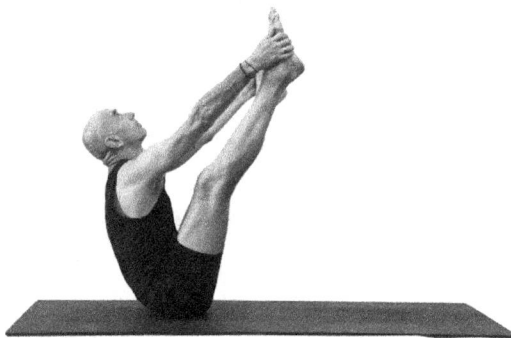

UPAVISTHA KONASANA B

1. Inhale up - raise the legs, don't release the hands, point the feet extending from the inner thighs, raise the chest, udiyana bandha engaged, look up. Take 6 breaths with sound. Dhristi up to space.

2. Exhale – release the legs

3. Inhale – enter the next asana.

Modification

If you can't catch the feet, catch the calf or ankles.

SUPTA KONASANA – RECLINING ANGLE POSE 2

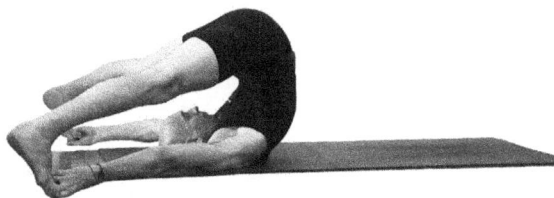

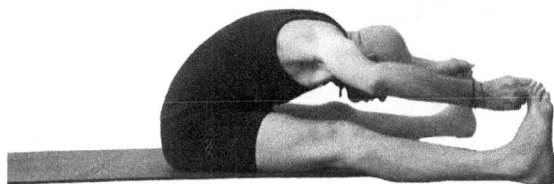

1. Inhale - lie down, exhale
2. Inhale - take the legs back over the head, catch the big toes, spread the legs. Take 6 breaths with sound. Dhristi nose.
3. Inhale - roll upto upright exhale down don't stop, don't release the feet.
4. Inhale - head up only, exhale there.
5. Inhale - lift up vinyasa.
6. Exhale - jump back to chaturanga plank position.
7. Inhale - lift the chest, urdha mukha (upward facing dog).
8. Exhale – raise the hips, ardha mukha (downward facing dog).

Modification

If you can't catch the feet, catch the calf or ankles.

SUPTA PADANGUSTHASANA – RECLINING BIG TOE POSE 2

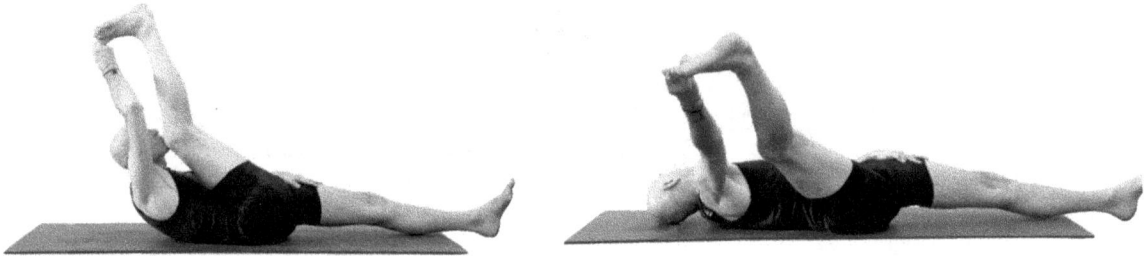

1. Inhale - jump through to sitting lie down, exhale.

2. Inhale - raise the right leg catch the big toe with the right hand, straight legs, left hand on thigh.

3. Exhale - chin to knee, Take 6 breaths with sound. Dhristi right big toe.

4. Inhale - head down, don't release the toe.

5. Exhale - take right leg out to the right side, straight leg, don't raise the left hip from the floor, look over the left shoulder, use the weight of the right leg to open the hip and increase the stretch. Take 6 breaths with sound. Dhristi into distance over left shoulder.

6. Inhale - bring leg back to centre, straight leg.

7. Exhale- chin to knee.

8. Inhale - head down.

9. Exhale - release the foot.

10. Inhale - raise the left leg catch the big toe, right hand on thigh.

11. Exhale - chin to knee, Take 6 breaths with sound. Dhristi left big toe.

12. Inhale - head down, don't release the toe,

13. Exhale - take left leg out to the left side, straight leg, look over the right shoulder, use the weight of the left leg to open the hip and increase the stretch. Take 6 breaths with sound. Dhristi into distance over right shoulder.

14. Inhale - bring leg back to centre, straight leg.

15. Exhale - chin to knee.

16. Inhale - head down.

17. Exhale - release the foot.

18. Inhale, chakrasana, - Backward roll into chaturanga, plank position, exhale.

19. Inhale - lift the chest, urdha mukha (upward facing dog).

20. Exhale - raise the hips, ardha mukha (downward facing dog).

Modification

If you can't catch with straight leg bend the knee slightly or use a towel to help intensify the stretch.

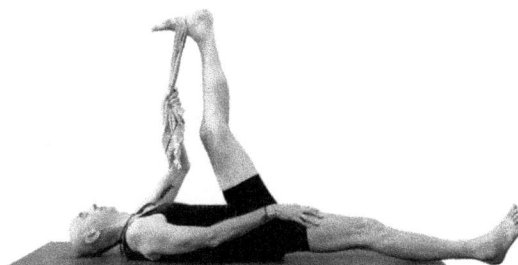

Chakrasana Modification

Backward roll over on one shoulder.

UBHAYA PADANGUSTHASANA – TWO FOOT POSE

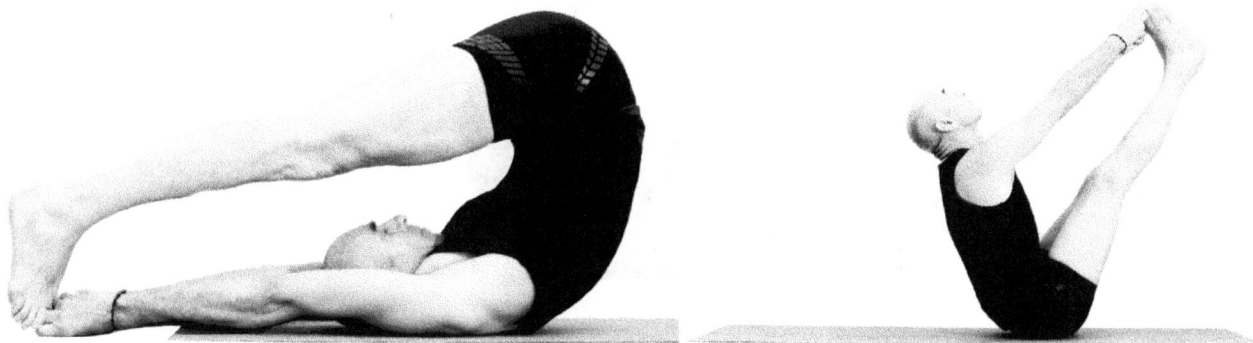

The next 2 asanas can be grouped together with vinyasa only entering and after finishing the set.

1. Inhale - jump through to sitting, lie down, exhale.
2. Inhale - take the legs back over the head, catch the big toes, exhale there.
3. Inhale – roll up into position, straight legs, point toes look up, extend the inner thighs, engage udiyana bandha, raise the chest, take 6 breaths with sound. Dhristi up to space.
4. Exhale – release the legs.

Continue in to the next asana

Modifications:

If you can't catch the toes, catch the ankles.

Bend the knees while coming back up.

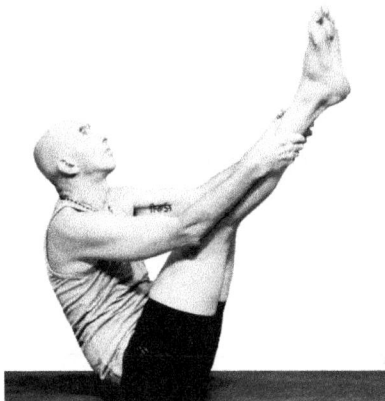

URDHVA MUKHA PACHIMATANASANA – UPWARD FACING INTENSE STRETCH 2

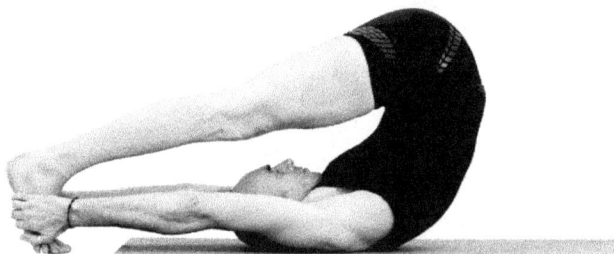

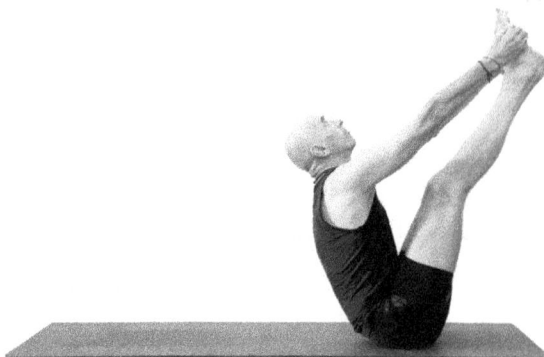

1. Exhale - lie down.

2. Inhale - take the legs back over the head, catch the outside of the feet, exhale there.

3. Inhale - roll up into position, straight legs, point the toes, extend the inner thighs, udiyana bandha engaged, raise the chest.

4. Exhale - chin to knees. Take 6 breaths with sound. Dhristi big toe

5. Inhale - straighten the arms, look up, exhale, take 6 breaths, Dhristi to the sky.

6. Inhale – up vinyasa

7. Exhale - jump back to chaturanga, plank position.

8. Inhale - lift the chest, urdha mukha (upward facing dog).

9. Exhale - raise the hips, ardha mukha (downward facing dog).

Modifications:

Bend the knees while coming back up.

If you can't catch the feet catch the ankles. See previous asana modification.

BACK BENDING SERIES OF ASANAS –NO VINYASA BETWEEN THE ASANAS.

DANURASANA - BOW POSE. X 3

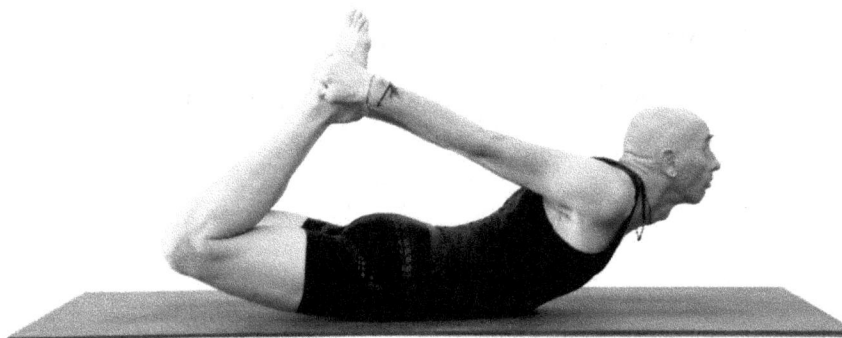

1. Inhale – lay down supine, exhale.
2. Inhale, catch the ankles, raise the chest, and the thighs, open heart, keep the knees and feet together, take 6 breaths, Dhristi nose
3. Exhale - down, don't release the ankles, take 3 breaths,
4. Inhale – up, raise the chest and the thighs, take 6 breaths, dhristi nose
5. Exhale - down, don't release the ankles, take 3 breaths,
6. Inhale – up, raise the chest and the thighs, take 6 breaths. Dhristi nose.
7. Exhale – release, move back to Balasana, child pose, take 6 breaths.

Continue to next asana.

USTRASANA

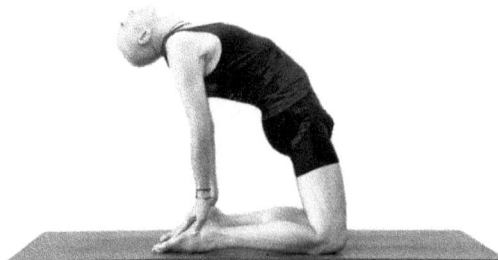

1. Inhale – come into kneeling position, top of the feet on the floor.

2. Exhale - lower the palms of the hands on to the soles of the feet, hips forward, open chest, take 9 breaths. Dhristi tip of the nose.

3. Inhale – up

4. Exhale – back to balasana position, child pose, take 6 breaths.

Continue to next asana.

Modification

Bring fingers to the heels or put your hands on the lower back, hips forward, lean back to comfortable position, 6 breaths.

LAGHUVAJRASANA

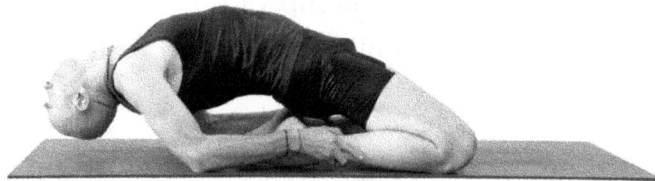

1. Inhale – come into kneeling position, top of the feet on the floor.

2. Exhale- lower the back down so the top of the head is on the floor, hands on thighs or calves.

3. Inhale – lift the hips, open chest, take 9 breaths. Dhristi third eye.

4. Inhale – come back up.

5. Exhale – back to balasana position, child pose, take 6 breaths.

6. Inhale – up vinyasa

7. Exhale – back to chaturanga, plank position.

8. Inhale – raise the chest, urdha mukha (upward facing dog)

9. Exhale – raise the hips, ardha mukha (downward facing dog).

URDHVA DANURASANA – LIFTED BOW POSE X 3

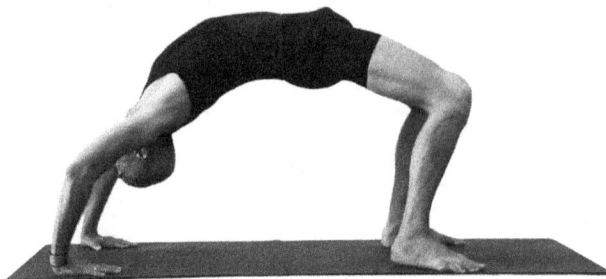

1. Inhale - jump through to sitting, lie down.

2. Exhale - bring the feet up towards the buttocks, same width as the shoulders, bring the arms over the head elbows bent, palms of the hands to the floor hands facing forward.

3. Inhale - raise the hips and the head from the floor, while pushing down with the hands and the feet, lifting from the pelvis, do not lift the heels. Take 6 breaths with sound. Dhristi nose

4. Exhale - down onto the top of the head, walk the hands in towards the shoulders. Inhale lift up, repeat, total 3 times.

5. Inhale - chakrasana backward roll into chaturanga plank position, exhale there.

6. Inhale - lift the chest, urdha mukha (upward facing dog).

7. Exhale - raise the hips, ardha mukha downward facing dog).

Modifications

If you can't lift up the torso on the first inhale, lift up onto the top of the head, exhale there, on next inhale lift all the way up .

If you can't lift all the way up into the final position, raise the knees, bring the ankles to the hands and lift up the hips, take 6 breaths exhale down, repeat 2 more times.

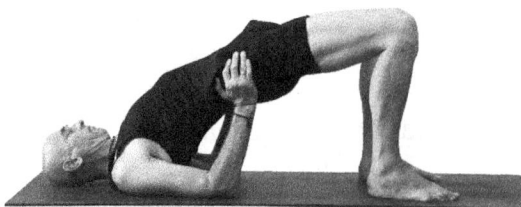

PACIMATTANASANA.

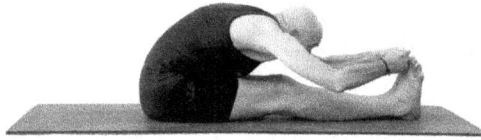

1. Inhale - jump through to sitting.
2. Exhale - fold forward catching the outside of the feet 8 breaths. Dhristi big toes.
3. Inhale – head up only, exhale there.
4. Inhale – up vinyasa
5. Exhale – back to chaturanga, plank position.
6. Inhale – raise the chest, urdha mukha (upward facing dog)
7. Exhale – raise the hips, ardha mukha (downward facing dog).

ASSISTED DROP BACK

We do assisted drop back depending on the student's ability and the time available, most people have the ability to do this with correct guidance.

1. Inhale – stand on the front of the mat, cross the hands on the chest, the teacher will support your hips, providing stability.
2. Exhale - fold backward, pushing forward with the hips, pelvic tilt, length in the spine open chest, bending from the lumber straight back, drop the neck, bend the knees
3. Inhale – Come back to upright, push down with the big toes strong legs, as the teacher pulls your hips forward.
4. Repeat 2 more times, total 3 times.
5. Inhale - Raise the arms, lengthen the spine,
6. Exhale - pushing forward with the hips, pelvic tilt, length in the spine open chest, bending from the lumber maintaining length in the spine, straight back, drop the neck, bend the knees, let the hands come to the floor Urdhva Danurasana, take 6 breaths, walk the hands closer to the feet on the inhale, catch the ankles if possible.
7. Inhale - Come back to upright, push down with the big toes strong legs, as the teacher pulls your hips forward
8. Exhale Samasthiti

Take pachimotanasana position and let the teacher bend you forwards to the maximum giving space back to the lumbar vertebrae, 8 breaths.

Forward bend after backward bend leads to safe back bending.

INVERSION SERIES OF ASANAS

SALAMBA SARVANGASANA - SHOULDERSTANDING POSE

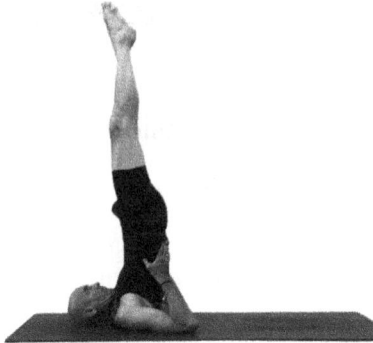

1. Inhale- jump through to sitting, lie down, exhale.
2. Inhale - raise the legs, lifting up onto the shoulders, hands placed on the lower back supporting the hips, feet together, strong legs, lifting the hips, hips forward feet back, udiyana bandha engaged, feet, hips, shoulders in a straight line. Take 18 breaths with sound. Dhristi nose.

HALASANA – PLOUGH POSE

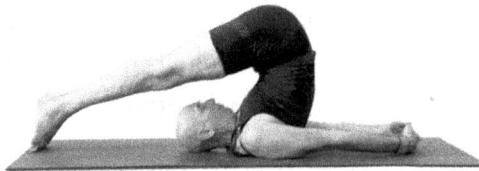

1. Exhale - lower straight legs to the floor behind the head, toes pointing back, top of the toes flat on the floor, Catch hands behind the back lengthen the arms. Take 9 breaths with sound. Dhristi nose.

Modification

Bend the legs slightly and support the hips if necessary.

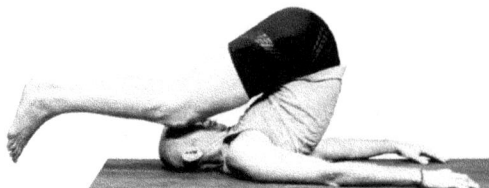

KARNA PIDASANA – EAR PRESSURE POSE

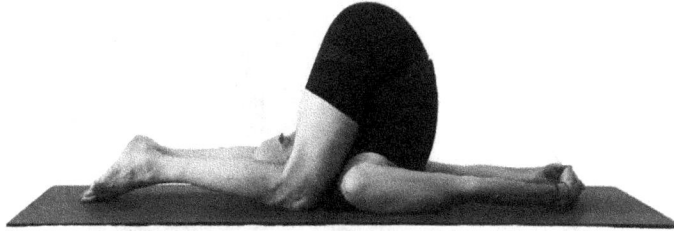

1. Exhale - bend the knees closing the ears with the knees, toes pointing back, top of the toes flat on the floor, hands remain behind the back, long arms. Take 9 breaths with sound. Dhristi nose.

Modification

Do not bring the knees down too far, lower to comfortable position while supporting the hips with the hands, take 9 breaths.

URDHVA PADMASANA – FLYING LOTUS POSE

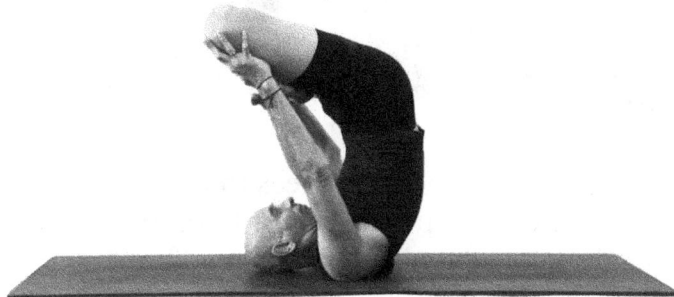

1. Inhale - raise the legs, take padmasana, drop the knees to 90 degrees, hands under the knees with straight arms, udiyana bandha engaged, take 9 breaths with sound. Dhristi nose.

Modification

If you can't do full lotus take half lotus position.

PINDASANA – EMBRYO POSE

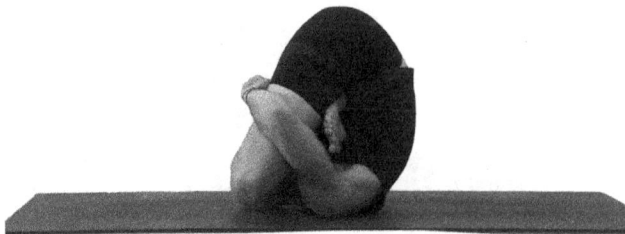

1. Exhale - drop the knees, catch the hands together around the legs, take 9 breaths with sound. Dhristi nose

Modification

Lotus or half lotus, if you can't catch the hands, stretch as far around the legs as possible.

MATSYASANA – FISH POSE

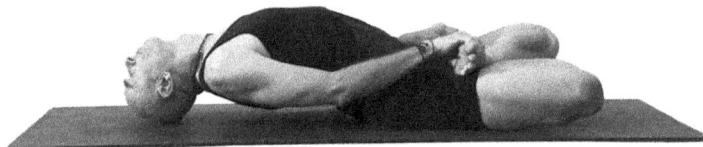

1. Exhale - release the hands, roll your knees to the floor without releasing padmasana, arch the back, lift the chest, open your heart, top of the head to the floor. Catch your feet with the hands, take 9 breaths with sound. Dhristi nose

Modification

If you are not in full lotus, half lotus or legs straight is acceptable.

UTTANA PADASANA – EXTENDED FOOT POSE

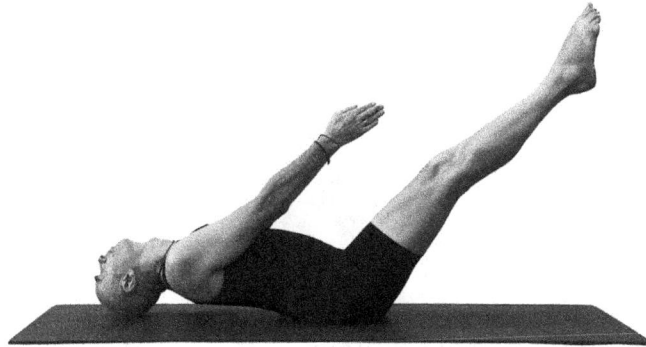

1. Inhale,- release padmasana, don't change the head position, lift straight legs to 45 degrees, raise the arms to 45 degrees, hands together. Take 9 breaths with sound. Dhristi nose.

2. Exhale release, lay down

3. Inhale chakrasana - backward roll into chaturanga, plank position, exhale

4. Inhale - lift the chest, urdha mukha (upward facing dog).

5. Exhale - raise the hips, ardha mukha (downward facing dog).

Modification

If you are can't lift legs and arms at the same time, try lifting them individually to build strength

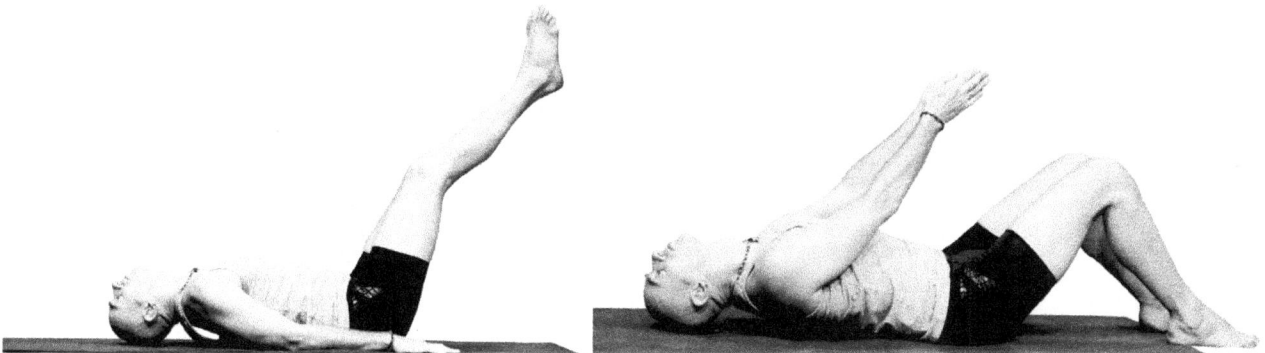

PINCHA MAYURASANA – FEATHER OF PEACOCK POSE.

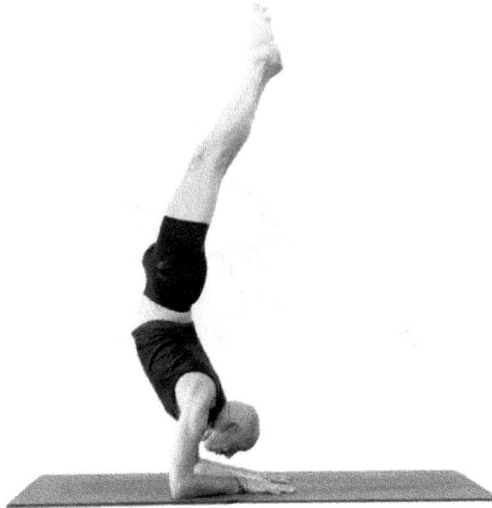

1. Inhale - drop the knees and take forearms to floor, palms of the hands down, elbows forearm width apart, head lifted from the floor.

2. Exhale – raise the hips, walk the feet forward,

3. Inhale – jump or lift the legs up, feet together, balancing on the forearms, lift from the shoulders, legs straight, udiyana bandha engaged, ankles, hips shoulders in a straight line, take 9 breaths. Dhristi nose.

4. Exhale – down, take balasana, (child pose) 6 breaths.

Modification

1. keep the head on the floor, balancing on forearms and head.

SIRSASANA – A- B-C. HEAD STANDING POSE.

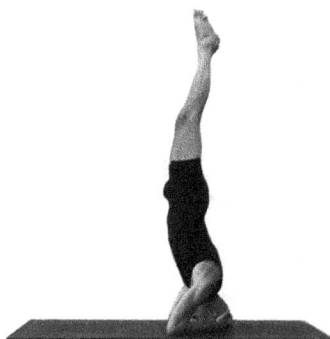

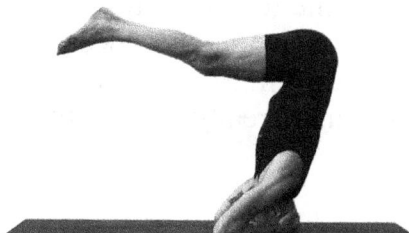

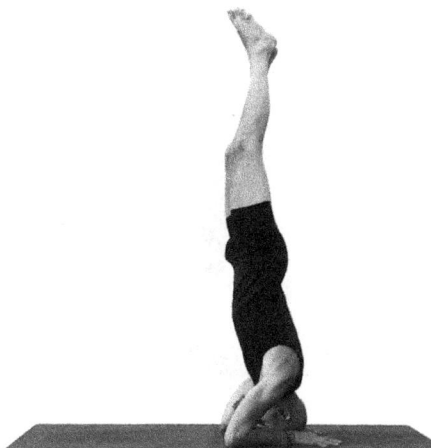

**(DO NOT PRACTICE SIRASANA IF YOU HAVE
GLAUCOMA, BP OR HEART CONDITION)**

1. Inhale - take position, make a triangle with the arms, elbows forearm width apart, clasp the fingers together wrists apart making a cup to place the head between the hands, head onto the floor, exhale there. The head rests on the floor about 2 inches above the hairline, (to find the right position for the head put the wrist crease on the tip of the nose, where the middle finger touches the top of the head this is the correct position)

2. Inhale - walk the feet forward hips above the shoulders, lift into position. Straight legs, feet together point the toes. Ankles, hips, shoulders, wrists should be in a straight line. Take 18 breaths with sound. Dhristi nose.

3. Exhale - drop the legs to 90 degrees strong legs, feet pointing forward, udiyana bandha engaged. Take 9 breaths with sound. Dhristi nose.

4. Inhale - lift the legs back up to sirasana position. Release the hands one at a time placing the palm down in front of the shoulders, 9 breaths with sound. Dhristi nose.

5. Exhale – lake the hands back to the head, lower the legs down to the floor slowly, take child pose. Take 8 breaths.

Modifications:

3 inhale, walk the feet and hips forward, bring one knee to chest, next bring bring the other knee to the chest, and breathe there. First get used to this position before trying to extend fully, this is still a headstand but with no fear. When you are ready, extend the legs.

SIRSASANA – D-E.

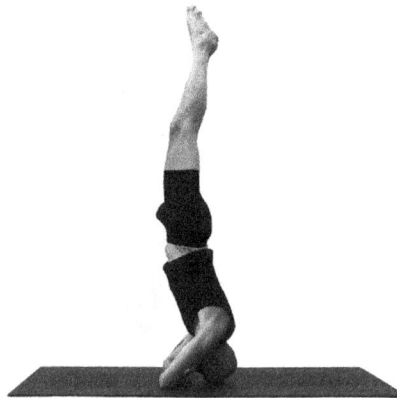

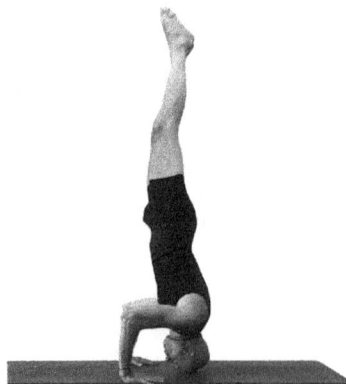

1. Inhale – take position, catch the elbows with the hands in front of your chest, place the head and forearms on the floor, exhale there.

2. Inhale - walk the feet forward hips above the shoulders, lift into position. Straight

legs, feet together point the toes. Ankles, hips, shoulders, head should be in a straight line. Take 9 breaths with sound. Dhristi nose.

3. Inhale – release the right hand, taking the hand back, palm down elbow at 90 degrees, exhale.

4. Inhale – release the left hand, taking the hand back, palm down elbow at 90 degrees, take 18 breaths with sound. Dhristi nose.

5. Exhale - lower legs down to the floor slowly, take child pose. Take 8 breaths.

6. Inhale - lift the chest, urdha mukha (upward facing dog).

7. Exhale - raise the hips, ardha mukha (downward facing dog).

Modifications:

If you are not able to take the transition into C and E, you can come down, takes the hands into position and come back up.

I consider Sirsasana A and E essential. A provides stability in mastering the pose where E works on strengthening the shoulders and preparing the neck for standing on the head alone without support.

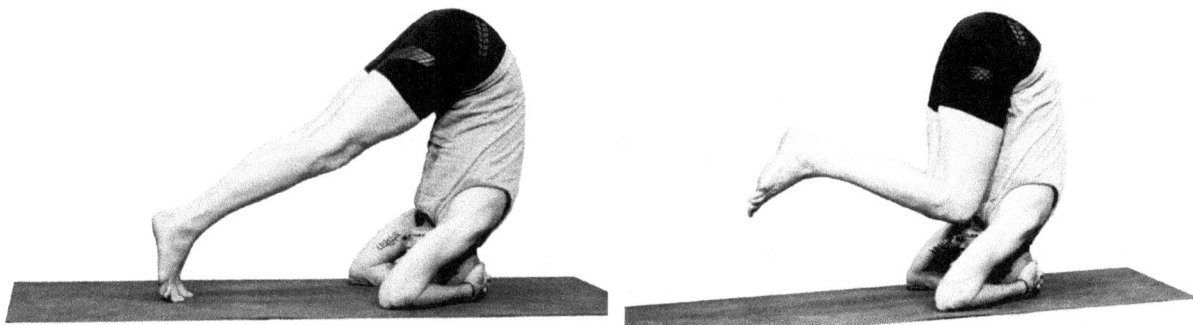

BADDHA PADMASANA – BOUND LOTUS POSE

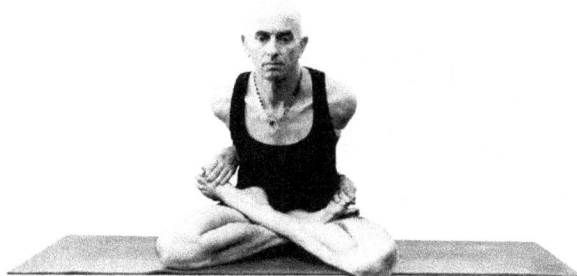

1. Inhale - jump through to sitting, exhale.

2. Inhale -take padmasana, bring the left hand round the back and catch the left big toe, take right hand round the back and catch the right big toe, raise the chest udiyana bandha engaged.

Modification

Catch the elbows instead of the feet, or use towels to catch the feet, exhale down.

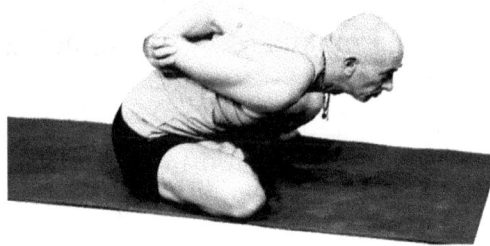

YOGA MUDRA A – SACRED SEAL

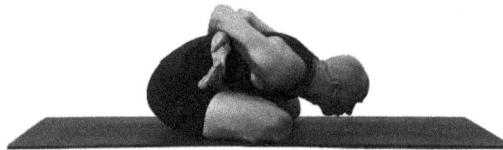

1. Exhale - bend forward, leading with the chest, lengthen the spine, chin to the floor. Take 9 breaths with sound. Dhristi nose

YOGA MUDRA B

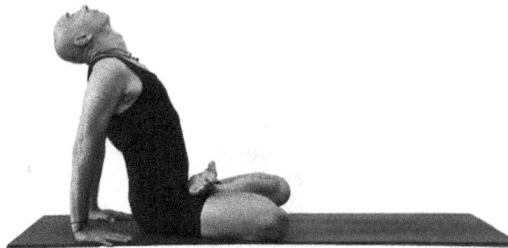

1. Inhale - come back up, take the hands back, about 12 inches behind the hips, raise the sternum and thoracic spine, udiyana engaged, relax the neck. Take 9 breaths with sound. Dhristi nose.

PADMASANA – FULL LOTUS POSE

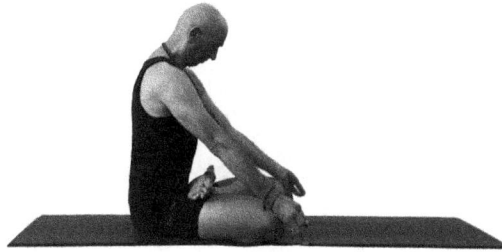

1. Inhale - raise the head and chest, take hand mudra. Straight back, drop the chin, all 3 bandhas engaged. Take 9 breaths with sound. Dhristi nose.

UTPLUTHI – SCALES POSE

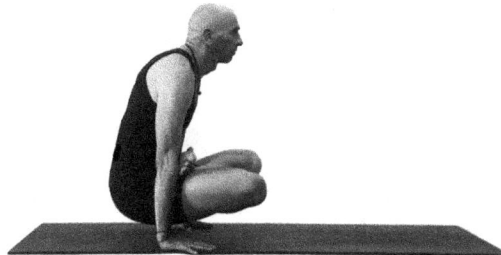

1. Inhale up - hands on the floor at the side of the waist, lift the knees, draw the body upwards from mula bandha, udiyana bandha engaged, don't drop the head, take 9 breaths with sound. Dhristi nose.

2. Exhale – down

3. Inhale - up vinyasa.

4. Exhale - jump back to chaturanga plank position.

5. Inhale - lift the chest, urdha mukha (upward facing dog).

6. Exhale raise the hips, ardha mukha (downward facing dog).

7. Inhale - jump through to sitting.

Modification

If you are not in full lotus, half lotus is acceptable, lift up, keeping the buttocks off the floor.

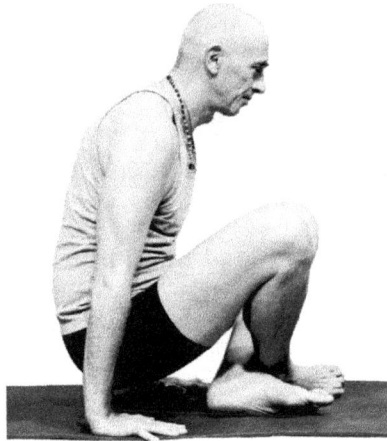

Bring the hands together in prayer position.

CLOSING MANTRA

Om

Yogena chitasya, padena vacham

Malam sharirasya, cha vaidyakena

Yopakarotham, pravaram muninaam

Patanjalim, pranjali ranatosmi.

Om Brahma Shakti Namaha

Om Brahma Shakti Namaha

Om Brahma Shakti Namaha

Om

Translation:

I bow with folded hands to the supreme sage Patanjali, who eradicated the impurity of mind with Yogashastra, impurity of speech with Vyakarana Mahabhashya, and impurity of body with Ayurveda literature.

Brahma is creation. Shakti is divine energy.

A NOTE ON SELF-PRACTICE.

When you do not have time for a full practice, rather than set unreasonable goals, it is better to do a modified practice than to do nothing. Unreasonable goals create the wrong mental balance, which may lead to someone giving up the practice altogether. Yoga should be enjoyable, the more you enjoy the practice and set reasonable goals the longer you will find time to get on your mat, thereby getting the maximum benefits for your body, mind and soul. "This is your practice, make your practice personal, feel the change".

Patanjali mentions in the Yoga Sutras that the 8 limbs of yoga are like a tree. Wisdom and spirituality develop in the same manner as a tree growing from a small seed, building a strong foundation of solid roots before reaching up to the sky. Different trees grow in different ways, some are small, others tall, thick, or thin but they are all trees developing together and completing their Dharma. Some grow quicker but they remain individual trees, there is no way to rush the growth.

You too can experience this growth and taste the fruits of the yoga tree. You can't hear someone's description to know the taste, you have to try it for yourself to enjoy its taste.

Through the practice of Brahma Shakti Vinyasa yoga you experience 7 of the 8 limbs of yoga (ashtanga yoga). Through regular practice you become more aware of your body, you eat more healthily and your mind becomes more peaceful. Yama and niyama begin to develop, Asana and Pranayama follow as you start to move and regulate your breathing. As you become more aware of the breath and link this with dristhi you are encouraged to turn inward and Prathyahara develops. As you improve, your mind becomes more focused and concentrated, Dharana develops and eventually meditation becomes automatic Dhyana. By practicing this way with patience and dedication you can hope to reach enlightenment. Yoga can be used as a way to simply keep fit and healthy but so many more subtle benefits are within, the only sure way to experience this is to practice with awareness.

The Full Brahma Shakti Vinyasa Yoga sequence detailed earlier takes around 90 minutes. Without Mantra and Pranayama (detailed in Section 5) which takes an extra 30 minutes.

In a studio class format, 90 minutes is allocated, starting with 12 minutes Mantra Meditation, 60 minutes asana and ending with Pranayama, I am giving four such class formats examples here but the teacher is free to change these formats so long as they still follow the sequence, and include all the asanas shown in **Bold Case** (below) in every practice, the teacher may also change to nine breaths in some asanas rather than the usual six but maintaining the asana practice at 60 minutes. Over the course of a six-day practice week the class format changes each day and ensures all asanas of the series are practiced several times throughout the week.

If time is limited do the asanas listed in bold text, this is a balanced short practice and can be completed easily, leaving time for Mantra and pranayama.

FULL PRACTICE 120 MINUTES

Start with Japa mantra meditation 12 minutes

Opening mantra

> **HANUMAN NAMASKAR x 2**
>
> **SURYA NAMASKAR A x 4**
>
> **SURYANAMASKAR B x 2**

standing - benefits tones muscles, massages internal organs

> **PADAN GUSTASANA**
>
> **PADA HASTASANA**
>
> UTTHITA TRIKONASANA A + B
>
> UTTHITA PARSVAKONASANA A + B
>
> PRASARITA PADOTTANASANA A + B + C +D
>
> PARSVOTTANASAN
>
> UTKATASANA (9)
>
> VIRABHADRASANA A + B

sitting- benefits tones muscles, massages internal organs

> **DANDASANA (9)**
>
> **PASCIMATTANASANA A + B**
>
> **ARDHA BADDHA PADMA PASCIMATTANASANA**
>
> TIRYANG MUKHA EKAPADA PASCIMATTANASANA
>
> JANUSIRSASANA A + B + C
>
> PARIGHASANA

MARICASANA A + B + C + D

ARDHA MATSYENDRASANA

GOMUKHASANA (9)

NAVASANA x 3 (9)

BADDHA KONASANA A&B

UPAVISTHA KONASANA

SUPTA KONASANA

SUPTA PADANGUSTHASANA - CHAKRASANA

UBHAYA PADANGUSTHASANA

URDHVA MUKHA PASCIMATTANASANA

back bending- maintains flexibility in the spine, release old emotions

DHANURASANA x 3

USTRASANA

LAGHU VAJRASANA

BALASANA

URDHVA DHANURASANA x 3 - CHAKRASANA

PASCIMATTANASANA

inversions- prevents aging, supplies blood to the brain.

SALAMBA SARVANGASANA (9)

HALASANA (9)

KARNA PIDASANA (9)

URDHVA PADMASANA (9)

PINDASANA (9)

MATSYASANA (9)

UTTANA PADASANA (9) - CHAKRASANA

PINCHA MAYURASANA (9)

SIRSASANA A (18) + B (9) + C (9) + D (9) + **E (18)**

finishing-

BADDHA PADMASANA - YOGA MUDRA A (9)

YOGA MUDRA B (9)

PADMASANA (9)

UTPLUTHIH (9)

Closing mantra.

Finish with pranayama 15 minutes

Shavasana

Asana in **Bold** must be in every practice option

Breaths in asana some (6) (9) or (18)

90 MINUTES PRACTICE OPTION ONE

Start with Japa mantra meditation 12 minutes

Opening mantra

HANUMAN NAMASKAR x 2

SURYA NAMASKAR A x 4

SURYANAMASKAR B x 2

standing - benefits tones muscles, massages internal organs

PADAN GUSTASANA

PADA HASTASANA

UTTHITA TRIKONASANA A + B

PARSVOTTANASAN

UTKATASANA (9)

VIRABHADRASANA A + B

sitting- benefits tones muscles, massages internal organs

DANDASANA (9)

PASCIMATTANASANA A + B

ARDHA BADDHA PADMA PASCIMATTANASANA

TIRYANG MUKHA EKAPADA PASCIMATTANASANA

JANUSIRSASANA A + C

MARICASANA A + C

ARDHA MATSYENDRASANA

NAVASANA x 3 (9)

BADDHA KONASANA A&B

UPAVISTHA KONASANA

SUPTA KONASANA

UBHAYA PADANGUSTHASANA

back bending- maintains flexibility in the spine, release old emotions

DHANURASANA x 3

USTRASANA

LAGHU VAJRASANA

BALASANA

PASCIMATTANASANA

inversions- prevents aging, supplies extra blood to the brain.

SALAMBA SARVANGASANA (9)

HALASANA (9)

KARNA PIDASANA (9)

URDHVA PADMASANA (9)

PINDASANA (9)

MATSYASANA (9)

UTTANA PADASANA (9) - CHAKRASANA

SIRSASANA A (18) + B (9) + C (9) + E (18)

finishing-

BADDHA PADMASANA - YOGA MUDRA A (9)

YOGA MUDRA B (9)

PADMASANA (9)

UTPLUTHIH (9)

Closing mantra.

Finish with pranayama 15 minutes

Shavasana.

90 MINUTES PRACTICE OPTION TWO

Start with Japa mantra meditation 12 minutes

Opening mantra

HANUMAN NAMASKAR x 2

SURYA NAMASKAR A x 4

SURYANAMASKAR B x 2

standing - benefits tones muscles, massages internal organs

PADAN GUSTASANA

PADA HASTASANA

UTTHITA PARSVAKONASANA A + B

PRASARITA PADOTTANASANA A + B + C +D

PARSVOTTANASAN

sitting- benefits tones muscles, massages internal organs

DANDASANA (9)

PASCIMATTANASANA A + B

ARDHA BADDHA PADMA PASCIMATTANASANA

JANUSIRSASANA A + B

PARIGHASANA

MARICASANA B + D

ARDHA MATSYENDRASANA

GOMUKHASANA (9)

NAVASANA x 3 (9)

BADDHA KONASANA A&B

SUPTA PADANGUSTHASANA - CHAKRASANA

URDHVA MUKHA PASCIMATTANASANA

back bending- maintains flexibility in the spine, release old emotions

DHANURASANA x 3

USTRASANA

LAGHU VAJRASANA

BALASANA

URDHVA DHANURASANA x 3 - CHAKRASANA

PASCIMATTANASANA

inversions- prevents aging, supplies extra blood to the brain.

PINCHA MAYURASANA (9)

SIRSASANA A (18) + B (9) + D (9) + E (18)

finishing-

BADDHA PADMASANA - YOGA MUDRA A (9)

YOGA MUDRA B (9)

PADMASANA (9)

UTPLUTHIH (9)

Closing mantra

Finish with pranayama 15 minutes

90 MINUTES PRACTICE OPTION THREE

Start with Japa mantra meditation 12 minutes

Opening mantra

> **HANUMAN NAMASKAR x 2**
>
> **SURYA NAMASKAR A x 4**
>
> **SURYANAMASKAR B x 2**

standing - benefits tones muscles, massages internal organs

> **PADAN GUSTASANA**
>
> **PADA HASTASANA**
>
> UTTHITA TRIKONASANA A + B
>
> PRASARITA PADOTTANASANA A + B + C +D
>
> UTKATASANA (9)
>
> VIRABHADRASANA A + B

sitting- benefits tones muscles, massages internal organs

> **DANDASANA (9)**
>
> **PASCIMATTANASANA A + B**
>
> **ARDHA BADDHA PADMA PASCIMATTANASANA**
>
> JANUSIRSASANA A + B + C
>
> PARIGHASANA
>
> GOMUKHASANA (9)
>
> **NAVASANA x 3 (9)**
>
> **BADDHA KONASANA A&B**
>
> UPAVISTHA KONASANA
>
> SUPTA KONASANA
>
> UBHAYA PADANGUSTHASANA

URDHVA MUKHA PASCIMATTANASANA

back bending- maintains flexibility in the spine, release old emotions

DHANURASANA x 3

USTRASANA

LAGHU VAJRASANA

BALASANA

PASCIMATTANASANA

inversions- prevents aging, supplies extra blood to the brain.

SALAMBA SARVANGASANA (9)

HALASANA (9)

KARNA PIDASANA (9)

URDHVA PADMASANA (9)

PINDASANA (9)

MATSYASANA (9)

UTTANA PADASANA (9) - CHAKRASANA

SIRSASANA A (18) + B (9) + D (9) + E (18)

finishing-

BADDHA PADMASANA - YOGA MUDRA A (9)

YOGA MUDRA B (9)

PADMASANA (9)

UTPLUTHIH (9)

Closing mantra

Finish with pranayama 15 minutes

Shavasana.

PRACTICE OPTION THREE

Start with Japa mantra meditation 1 minutes

Opening mantra

> **HANUMAN NAMASKAR x 2**
>
> **SURYA NAMASKAR A x 4**
>
> **SURYANAMASKAR B x 2**

standing - benefits tones muscles, massages internal organs

> **PADAN GUSTASANA**
>
> **PADA HASTASANA**
>
> UTTHITA TRIKONASANA A + B
>
> PRASARITA PADOTTANASANA A + B + C +D
>
> UTKATASANA (9)
>
> VIRABHADRASANA A + B

sitting- benefits tones muscles, massages internal organs

> **DANDASANA (9)**
>
> **PASCIMATTANASANA A + B**
>
> **ARDHA BADDHA PADMA PASCIMATTANASANA**
>
> JANUSIRSASANA A + B + C
>
> PARIGHASANA
>
> GOMUKHASANA (9)
>
> **NAVASANA x 3 (9)**
>
> **BADDHA KONASANA A&B**
>
> UPAVISTHA KONASANA
>
> SUPTA KONASANA
>
> UBHAYA PADANGUSTHASANA

URDHVA MUKHA PASCIMATTANASANA

back bending- maintains flexibility in the spine, release old emotions

DHANURASANA x 3

USTRASANA

LAGHU VAJRASANA

BALASANA

PASCIMATTANASANA

inversions- prevents aging, supplies extra blood to the brain.

SALAMBA SARVANGASANA (9)

HALASANA (9)

KARNA PIDASANA (9)

URDHVA PADMASANA (9)

PINDASANA (9)

MATSYASANA (9)

UTTANA PADASANA (9) - CHAKRASANA

SIRSASANA A (18) + B (9) + D (9) + E (18)

finishing-

BADDHA PADMASANA - YOGA MUDRA A (9)

YOGA MUDRA B (9)

PADMASANA (9)

UTPLUTHIH (9)

Closing mantra

Finish with pranayama 15 minutes

Shavasana.

90 MINUTES PRACTICE OPTION FOUR

Start with Japa mantra meditation 12 minutes

Opening mantra

HANUMAN NAMASKAR x 2

SURYA NAMASKAR A x 4

SURYANAMASKAR B x 2

standing - benefits tones muscles, massages internal organs

PADAN GUSTASANA

PADA HASTASANA

UTTHITA PARSVAKONASANA A + B

PRASARITA PADOTTANASANA A + B + C +D

UTKATASANA (9)

VIRABHADRASANA A + B

sitting- benefits tones muscles, massages internal organs

DANDASANA (9)

PASCIMATTANASANA A + B

ARDHA BADDHA PADMA PASCIMATTANASANA

TIRYANG MUKHA EKAPADA PASCIMATTANASANA

JANUSIRSASANA A + C

MARICASANA A + C

ARDHA MATSYENDRASANA

GOMUKHASANA

NAVASANA x 3 (9)

BADDHA KONASANA A&B

SUPTA KONASANA

SUPTA PADANGUSTHASANA - CHAKRASANA

URDHVA MUKHA PASCIMATTANASANA

back bending- maintains flexibility in the spine, release old emotions

DHANURASANA x 3

USTRASANA

LAGHUVAJRASANA

URDHVA DHANURASANA x 3 - CHAKRASANA

PASCIMATTANASANA

Inversions- prevents aging, supplies extra blood to the brain.

PINCHA MAYURASANA (9)

SIRSASANA A (18) + B (9) + C (9) + E (18)

finishing-

BADDHA PADMASANA - YOGA MUDRA A (9)

YOGA MUDRA B (9)

PADMASANA (9)

UTPLUTHIH (9)

Closing mantra

Finish with pranayama 15 minutes

Shavasana.

SECTION 5: THE PRACTICE, PRANAYAMA.

Definition of Pranayama: Prana means life force or breath sustaining the body; Ayama translates as "to extend or draw out."

Ten reasons why breathing exercises are beneficial:

1. Improves brain function
2. Soothes the nervous system
3. Cleans the lungs
4. Calms the mind
5. Enhances relaxation
6. Improves sleep
7. Boosts energy
8. Enhances rest
9. Merges the left and right side of the brain
10. Prepares the mind and body for meditation.

THE SCIENCE OF BREATH

Most people use only a small percentage of their lung capacity. Usually their shoulders are dropped and closed, which restricts the lungs from expanding fully, resulting in the lungs losing their elasticity.

There are three main ways to describe how people breathe.

1. Clavicular breathing, using the upper portion of the lungs is the worst, maximum effort is made on the inhale but minimum oxygen is obtained.
2. Abdominal breathing is the most common, using only the lower portion of the lungs.
3. Optimal breathing or full yoga breath is the most efficient, when we inhale from the

bottom of the lungs and allow the oxygen to fill the lungs gradually, expanding the chest and reaching the top of the lungs maximizing our intake of oxygen.

To experience full yogic breath, sit or stand erect with chest and shoulders open. Breathe in slowly from the bottom of the lungs, drawing the air past the stomach expanding the rib cage and into the upper portion of the lungs, exhale in the same manner, expelling all the air. This is the most efficient way to breathe.

A lesson can be learned from the animal kingdom, dogs have a life expectancy of around 10 to 14 years; their breathing is short and rapid, where as a elephant has long slow breath and have a life span of 80 to 100 years.

"Long breath, long life, short breath, short life".

Breathing is the single most important thing that we do, we can live without food for around one month, we can live without water for around two weeks, if we do not breathe we die within 5 to 7 minutes.

Pranayama is a form of breath control. It is a conscious technique of inhalation, retention of breath, exhalation and suspension of breath in exhalation.

In Pranayama the mind and the consciousness are controlled, which in turn optimizes all the functions of the body preventing disease.

Advanced pranayama techniques should be learnt under the guidance of an experienced teacher as incorrect practice can bring disease to the body, this is confirmed in the yoga shastra's.

Pranayama teaches us how to reduce the respiratory and heart rate, when the respiratory rate is reduced, the metabolic rate of the body is also reduced, the cells are rested and relaxation happens.

There are many types of pranayama each having a different effect on the body, all types of pranayama work on a proven physiological basis.

Normal resting respiratory rate in a adult is 12 to 16 breaths per minute, the reduction of respiratory rate to around 10 per minute through yoga and pranayama is optimal and has a noticeable effect on our whole system.

THE BENEFICIAL EFFECTS OF PRANAYAMA

RESPIRATORY SYSTEM

1. Pranayama, conscious deep breathing, allows the cells to become nourished with

oxygen, allowing more inflow of oxygen to the blood which is processed by the heart and pumped to the extremities of the body

2. Elasticity of the lungs is maintained through to old age, with vital capacity increased and dead space in the lungs decreased.

3. The alveoli are exercised which promotes better excretion of toxins and gasses.

4. Ventilation of the sinuses promoting good drainage.

5. Healthy movement of the diaphragm which is the major muscle used in breathing.

6. Massages the abdominal organs improving blood supply to those areas.

CARDIOVASCULAR SYSTEM

1. Due to constant change in the heart chamber size, the cardiac wall is exercised without strain, ensuring complete filling and emptying of the heart chamber.

2. The heart rate is reduced.

3. As more capillaries are opened up, microcirculation is enhanced, increasing the supply of nutrients to the cells, increasing their longevity. This all happens without increasing the pulse rate or blood pressure.

4. The most important effect is the washing away of free radicals (unstable atoms that damage cells) that damage the heart.

DIGESTIVE SYSTEM

1. Pranayama techniques stimulate the taste buds and salivary glands, improving digestive absorption and eliminatory function.

2. The stomach liver and gall bladder are massaged improving their function.

SKIN

1. Pranayama helps maintain healthy secretory functions of the skin.

2. It promotes increased blood flow to the dermis.

ENDOCRINE SYSTEM

All the endocrine glands are toned in pranayama.

NERVOUS SYSTEM

This is where the effects of pranayama have the most beneficial effect.

1. The awareness of the mind on the breath and its rhythm quietens the entire body and the mind becomes calm.
2. Pranayama enables mental peace, improving the ability to cope with stress.
3. As the nerves are soothed, cerebral circulation improves.

GENERAL BENEFITS

1. The body becomes lean strong and healthy.
2. Fat is reduced.
3. Pranayama prevents and cures disease.
4. The Nadis are purified.
5. The mind is prepared for, pratyahara, dharana and dhyana (the 3 stages of meditation)
6. Constant practice arouses spiritual strength, happiness, peace of mind and leads us towards samadhi.

Hatha Yoga Pradipika says: "the mind is the controller of the body but the breath is the controller of the mind"

HAND MUDRA.

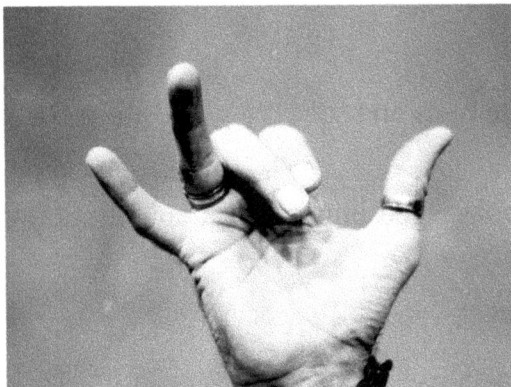

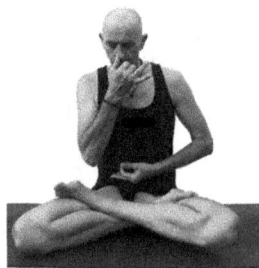

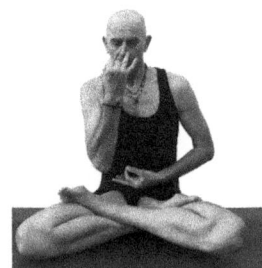

ALTERNATE NOSTRIL BREATHING WITH BANDHA L5-R5

1. Sit in a comfortable position with legs crossed and back straight.
2. Make a hand mudra with right hand (as shown in photo), close the right nostril with

the thumb, exhale through the left nostril for a count of 8, engage moola bandha and inhale through the left nostril for a count of 8.

3. Close left nostril with ring finger and exhale through the right nostril drawing in udiyana for count of 8.

4. Close the right nostril with the thumb, engage moola bandha inhale left nostril to count of 8.

5. Repeat this sequence 4 more times, total 5 rounds.

6. Repeat opposite side, close left nostril with ring finger, engage moola bandha inhale through right nostril to count of 8.

7. Close right nostril with thumb, exhale through left, drawing in udiyana bandha to count of 8.

8. Repeat 4 more times, total 5.

Gradually increase the number of rounds when you feel ready (maximum of 20 rounds).

BENEFITS OF ALTERNATE NOSTRIL AND BANDHA

- It regulates the respiratory system, balances and cleanses the left and right sides of the brain.

- It enhances bandha awareness and muscle function.

KAPALABHATI 50 ROUNDS 5 TIMES.

1. Sit in a comfortable position with legs crossed and back straight, do not engage bandhas.

2. Inhale fully.

3. Draw in the stomach forcing the exhalation, repeat 50 times. Concentrate on the exhalation, inhalation happens automatically.

4. Release, normal breathing 10 breaths

5. Repeat 4 more times, total 5.

BENEFITS OF KAPALABHATI.

- Kapalabhati generates heat in the body dissolving toxins and other waste matter, it improves function of the kidneys and liver, it removes stress from the eyes and enhances blood circulation and digestion, it tones the body giving better physical state.

- Kapalabhati is one of the 6 Kriyas, 'Hindu cleanses' mentioned later in the book.

NADI SHODHANA – ALTERNATE NOSTRIL BREATHING - 10 ROUNDS, EXHALE 8, INHALE 4

Nadi Shodhana is a nerve cleansing pranayama

1. Sit in a comfortable position with legs crossed and back straight, engage moola bandha and uddiyana bandha throughout.
2. Make a hand mudra with the right hand, close the right nostril with the thumb of the right hand; exhale from the left nostril for 8 silent counts
3. Inhale for only 4 counts through the same left nostril
4. Close left nostril with ring finger, exhale from the right nostril for 8 counts
5. Inhale for 4 counts through the right nostril
6. Close the right nostril with the thumb; exhale for 8 counts from left nostril.

Repeat steps 2 to 6 (1 round) ten times. Gradually increase the number of rounds when you feel ready (maximum of 20 rounds).

If you cannot exhale to the count of 8 do 6 exhalations and 3 inhalations. With practice your lungs will get stronger and you will be able do the full count of 8 or more.

In this exercise, remember to exhale for twice the length of the inhalation.

This technique can be used at the end of your yoga practice or any time you feel tension throughout the day, cleansing the left thinking side of the brain.

By concentrating on manipura chakra while practicing nadi shodhana it will help to awaken the dormant kundalini energy and encourage it to rise through the chakra centres.

BENEFITS OF NADI SHODHANA.

- It infuses the body with oxygen clearing and releasing toxins.

- It reduces stress and anxiety, calms and rejuvenates the nervous system.

- It helps to balance hormones.

- It alleviates respiratory allergies that cause hay fever, sneezing and wheezing.

- Balances the left side and right side of the brain, left side thinking and logic right side creative, imagination, memory.

SAMA VRITTI - EQUAL INHALE, EQUAL EXHALE X 10,

1. Remain in a comfortable position with legs crossed and back straight, all three bandha engaged, take hand mudra, hands on knees.

2. Inhale into top of the lungs to count of 8.

3. Exhale all the way to the base to count of 8.

4. Repeat 10 times.

5. Release, normal breathing.

BENEFITS OF SAMA VRITTI,

- The three doshas - vata, kapha and pitta - are regularized; blood pressure and diabetes can be cured completely.

- Diseases of the muscular system are cured and it is beneficial in arthritis, flatulence, varicose veins, acidity and sinusitis.

- Thought becomes positive and you are able to overcome tension, anger, worry, anxiety and it improves the memory.

- It increases oxygen supply throughout the body, improving blood circulation.

- Relieves fever, eye and ear problems, controls obesity and streamlines the metabolism.

- It relaxes and calms the brain.

A NOTE ON SELF-PRACTICE

Self practice can be difficult to maintain but you should persevere and find your own self practice, especially if sometimes you are unabe to attend class, it is a practice which fits your needs at that moment, It is your choice what asanas to do within the sequence, to take as many breaths as you want in asana and chose when you want to do vinyasa, enjoy this special time, create balance with the meditation and the pranayama and look forward to a beautiful day.

SECTION 6: JUMP THROUGH, JUMP BACK VINYASA.

I refer to vinyasa in this context as both the transition into and the exit from asana.

JUMPING THROUGH

From downward facing dog position:

- Inhale - bandhas engaged, gazing point should be in front of your hands, ahead of where you intend to land your feet. Bend the knees and jump the hips with a upward trajectory, If you lead with the hips, the legs will follow. When you reach the top of the jump, tuck the sitting bones under, lowering and crossing the legs, bringing them through the hands to sitting position.

Some people come through with straight legs, some people with crossed legs, both are correct, the key is strong bandha.

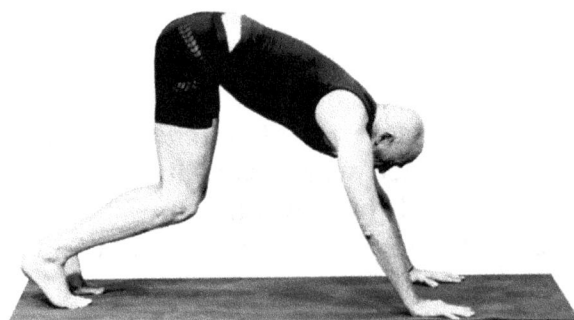

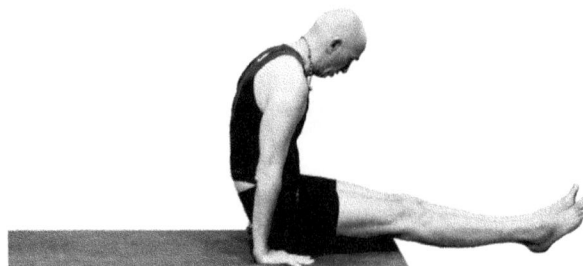

Modifications:

If you can't jump the legs through, don't worry; your arms are not too short! In time with dedicated practice and bandha, it will come. Try this:

• Inhale - jump the feet between the hands as far as possible, now continue to walk through the hands without raising the wrists off the floor, straighten the legs then lower down.

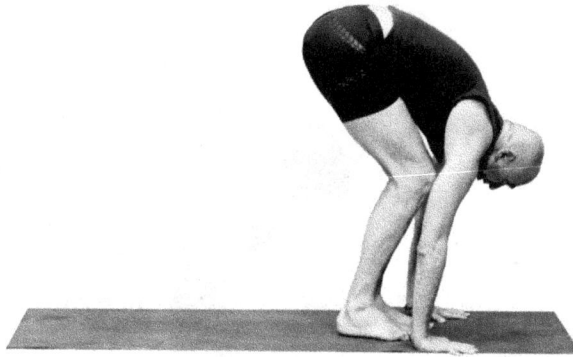

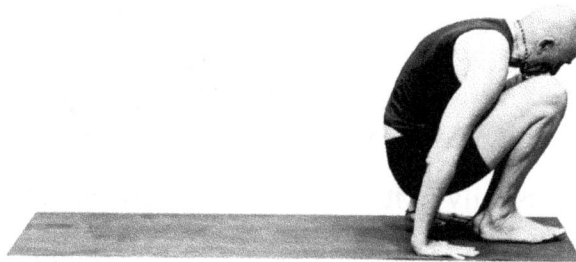

Remember to look ahead of where you expect your feet to land.

If the jump through is too difficult you can walk forward from downward facing dog, trying to bring the feet through the hands before sitting.

ONE-YEAR CHALLENGE

Get 2 books each with around 300 to 400 pages, place your hands on the books and jump through as if you were using blocks. Each day rip out one page from each book and within a year you will be jumping through without assistance.

You can also use the books to learn the 'lift up', drawing the energy up with bandha as in vinyasa and Utplutih.

JUMPING BACK

As you finish the asanas from sitting position.

1. Inhale – lift up, bring the hands to the floor, legs crossed to allow jump back.
2. Chatwari exhale - jump or walk back into chaturanga, plank position.
3. Inhale - raise the chest Ardha Mukha (upward facing dog).
4. Exhale - raise the hips Urdha Mukha (downward facing dog).

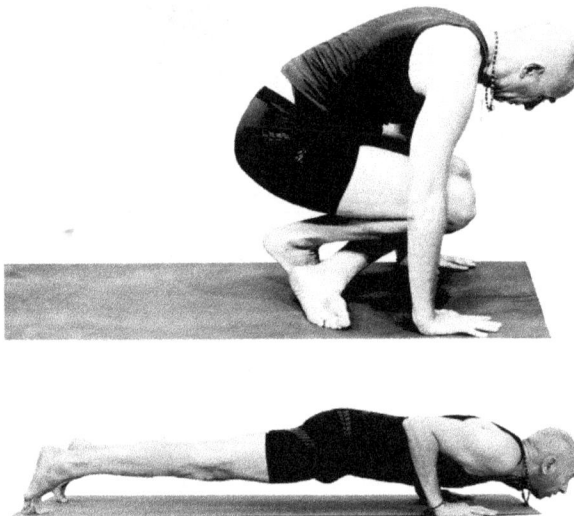

Advanced practitioners will usually exit vinyasa the following way.

1. Inhale – lift up, balancing on the hands, legs crossed above the ankle, knees to chest.
2. Chatwari exhale - lower the head towards the floor without touching the floor with your feet, Swing your legs back and through the arms, straight legs to Chaturanga Dandasana (plank position).

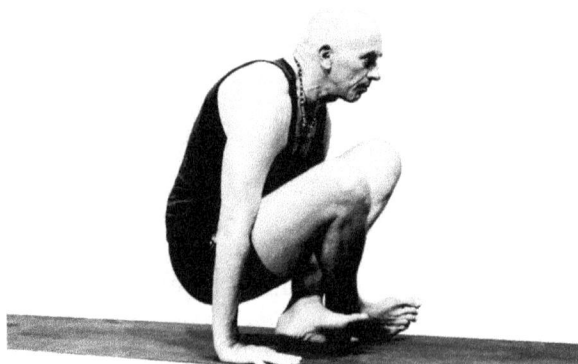

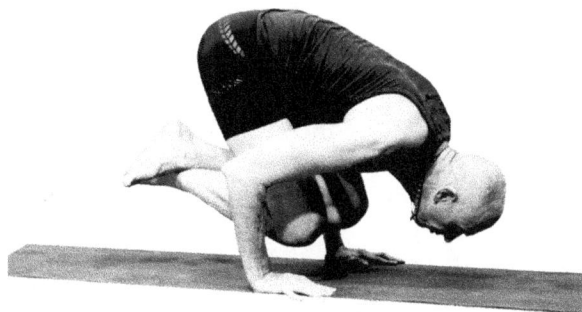

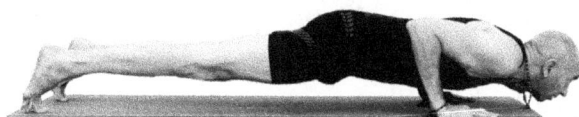

Again the secret to this vinyasa movement and transfer of weight is bandha. Keep checking your bandha. Strong bandha; light body. ''practice, practice all is coming''

SECTION 7: CHAKRASANA.

1. Lying down on the back, bring the hands behind the shoulders, palms down fingers pointing forward towards the feet.

2. Inhale - Bring your legs back, knees to chest and over the head, press the hands down into the floor and let the momentum and the weight of the hips take you back.

3. Exhale - as you land in chaturanga, plank position.

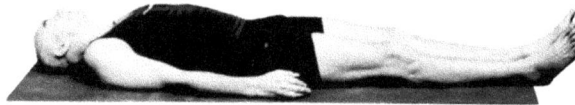

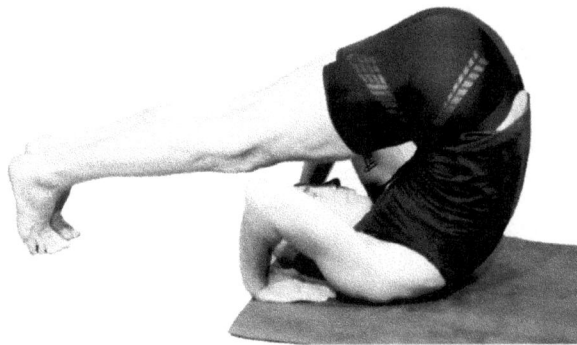

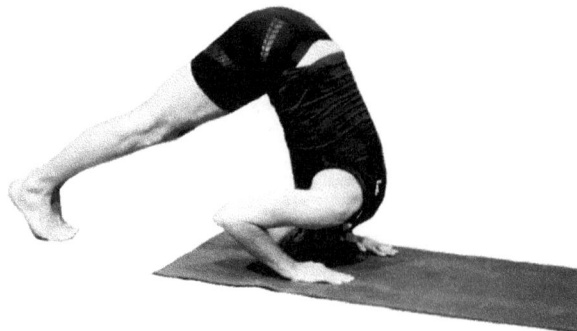

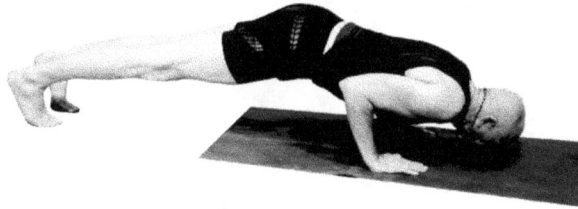

Modification

- Bring the hands behind the shoulders, fingers pointing back.

- Inhale - Bring your legs back, knees to chest and over the head, press the hands down into the floor and roll over on one shoulder.

By practicing this way you will learn to experience the 'lift' from pressing down with the hands, eventually learning to lift and roll back over the head without fear of hurting your neck.

SECTION 8: PADMASANA.

Padmasana is often the first big challenge when most people start yoga. Through the western habit of sitting in chairs our hips are often very closed. I see many students in my workshops who could very easily sit in padmasana but they do not know the correct technique to attain it.

1. Sit with straight legs and straight back, bandhas engaged. Inhale raise the right knee pulling the heel as close to your buttocks as possible safely stretching the knee.

2. Exhale let the right knee fall out to the side opening the hip. 2 padmasana mod

3. Inhale bring the right heel up towards the naval, keep the foot pointing forward engaged, 3 padmasana mod

4. Exhale, keeping the foot as high as possible on the thigh, allow the knee to relax down, open the calf muscle 4 padmasana mod

5. Inhale bring the left leg into position.

When in the final position, maintaining length in the spine push forward with the pelvic spine to set the natural arch, engage moola bandha and udiyana bandha.

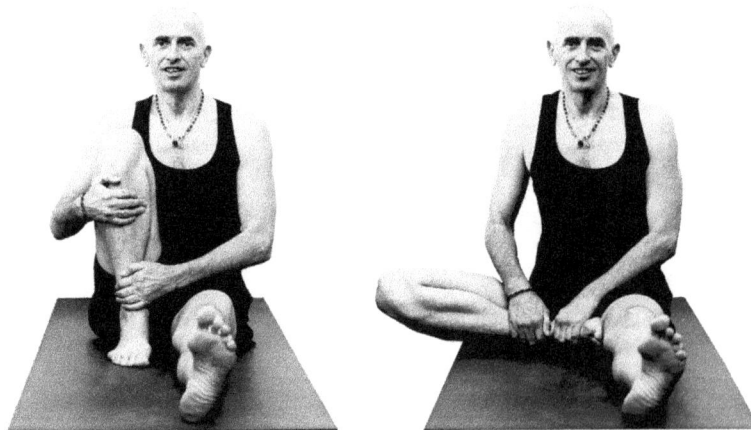

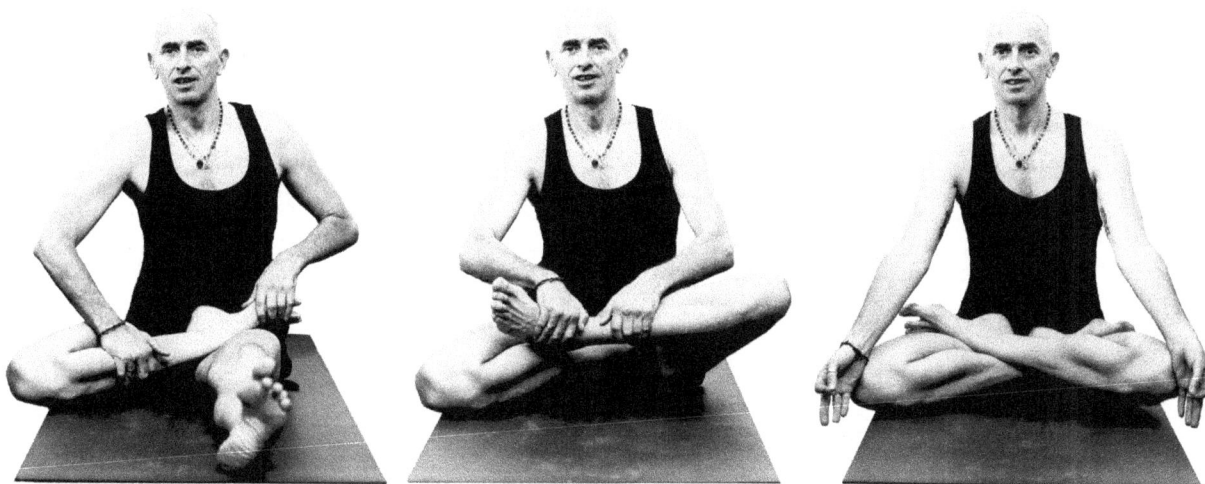

Hold padmasana comfortably with awareness on the breath.

If you feel too much discomfort, release and try again, slowly increase the length of time you can sit each day without strain, over time it will feel natural to sit this way.

SECTION 9: THE 8 LIMBS OF YOGA.

1. Yama: The five external moral restraints.

    Ahimsa : Non violence.

    Sathya: Truthfulness, non lying.

    Bramacharya: Control of sexual desires.

    Asthya: No stealing/ jealousy.

    Aparigraha; Non-possessive, freedom from desire.

2. Niyama: The five internal observances, self discipline.

    Saucha: Cleanliness, purity.

    Santosha: Contentment.

    Tapas: Austerity, self discipline.

    Swadhya: Self study and study of sacred texts.

    Ishwara Pranidhana, awareness of the supreme.

3. Asana: Posture.

4. Pranayama: Breath control/ vital energy.

5. Prathyahara: Turning inward, withdrawal of the senses.

6. Dharana: Concentration calming the distractions of the mind.

7. Dhyana: Meditation, awareness without focus.

8. Samadhi: Spiritual enlightenment.

SECTION 10: INDIAN PHILOSOPHY 'A GLIMPSE'

HISTORY OF MANKIND

In Indian philosophy, the history of mankind begins with a search for comforts to lead a happy life. It is the desire of every human being to have a happy and pleasant life with all comforts. Comforts are attained only through effort.

A person comes across other people, soon he becomes part of a group showing care and concern for others, he establishes a relationship and lives with others, he has established love, care and concern with material comforts. Unknowingly he has developed attachment to people and material comforts. In this bondage of attachment he fails to enjoy the comforts gained by hard work and struggle, they are only materials that do not have feeling. Eventually they fail to give delight. The delights are not in the item they are in the enjoyer. A pleasant mind alone can make the item pleasant.

IDENTIFICATION

Often we claim, 'this is my house' 'my car' 'my clothes' etc. but we fail to identify 'Who I Am'. Is it my name or form that are my identification? Often our identification goes with the objects or things that we possess, attaining satisfaction is only possible through self-realization.

VEDIC PHILOSOPHY: ANCIENT HINDU SYSTEMS OF THOUGHT.

Through the ages Indian philosophy has developed and reached the highest level. There are six main schools of thought honored by Vedic experts.

1. Samkhya

2. Yoga

3. Nyaya

4. Vaisheshika

5. Vedanta

6. Mimamsa

Samkhya philosophy regards the universe has having two realities, prakrithi/matter and purusa/consciousness. The existence of God is not considered by samkhya and considers the Vedas as a reliable source of knowledge, some people say it is an atheistic philosophy. Samkhya is known for its theory of the three gunas: sattva, rajas and tamas. It states that all matter has 3 gunas but in different proportions, these gunas determine the character of someone or something and influence the progress of life.

Yoga is one of the six schools of Hindu philosophy and is closely related to Samkhya. Yoga philosophy believes in systematic study to better one's self physically, mentally and spiritually and it has influenced all other schools of Indian philosophy. The sutras of Patanjali is the most important text of yoga philosophy.

Nyaya's most significant contribution to Hindu philosophy was the development of logic and methodology and relies on reliable means of gaining knowledge, perception, evidence, reasoning, comparison and testimony from reliable sources. Stating that human suffering results from wrong knowledge, while correct knowledge is discovery and overcoming delusion by understanding the true nature of self, soul and reality.

Vaisheshika In its early stage was an independent philosophy with its own logic but over time it became closely linked to Nyaya philosophy. Like Buddhism vaisheshika accepts only two means to knowledge - perception and inference, both consider their respective scriptures as indisputable. According to Vaisheshika knowledge and liberation were only achievable by complete understanding of the world of experience.

Vedanta is based on the philosophies contained in the Upanishads, it regards neither dualism nor non dualism as the absolute truth, adopting ideas from yoga philosophy and Nyaya. Vedanta has a historic influence on Hinduism stating that our real nature is the divine and exists in everyone but is often clouded by our own ignorance.

Mimamsa is believed to be the oldest of the six schools and focuses on Hindu rituals as a means to attaining enlightenment. It states there is no reason to believe that God exists or does not exist and everything in the universe came and continues to come through natural processes and believes in the reality of the soul and the external world.

Indian Philosophy recognizes four important texts

1. Brahmasuthra.

2. Bhagavad-Gita.

3. Upanishads.

4. Yoga sutras.

Brahmasuthra provides a definite description of the philosophical concept in definitions. The sentences are compact and clear, they provide complete meaning and understanding.

Bhagavad-Gita describes personality and guides us on how to develop personality. It is a discourse between Krisna the teacher and Arjuna the student, set on the battlefield of the Mahabharata war.

Upanishads are also called the Vedanta, each Veda has a set of Upanishads. The main topic is the understanding of:

- Jeeva - life or person.

- Jagath - the world.

- Eshwara - the supreme power.

We see an elaborate discussion on Atman, the soul, and Brahma, super natural energy. The verses give guidelines on ideal living.

Yoga sutras of Patanjali, contains 4 chapters and describes in short sentences how to better one's self physically, mentally and spiritually.

KLESHAS OR CAUSES OF SUFFERING

Human beings in search of happiness have always been looking outside themselves instead of internally. There are a few obstacles that cause much suffering. Yogis should make a conscious effort to overcome them.

1. Avidya - ignorance.
2. Asmita - ego.
3. Raga - attachment.
4. Dwesha - aversion.
5. Abhinivesha - intense desire for life.

Avidya, ignorance, is one of the main causes of suffering, Patanjali calls this the prominent cause of suffering and influences all other cause of suffering. The aim of yoga is to get liberation from the bondage of the mundane world, but as long as the person remains ignorant, liberation remains far away.

The person who is in Avidya tries to see immortality in mortals, eternal in the non-eternal, purity in the impure, pleasure in pain, he finds delight in the objective world. Patanjali says "the objects that give sensual pleasure will not last long"

Asmita, the ego, is a shroud that causes us to forget the limitations and scope of our identity.

This is when we can fall into the trap of having an ego that is too big or powerful which leads to conflict in many aspects of our life causing anger and suffering.

Raga, attachment, according to Vedanta the entire objective world is non-eternal and some-day will become extinct. The yoga student should realize that the world made up of materials is perishable, even the body made up of muscles, bones and tissue is perishable. This material world is non-eternal, only the soul 'Atman' is eternal.

Dwesha, aversion is an emotional response that negatively influences our perception of the world. Preferences are born out of our previous experiences resulting in likes and dislikes. Being influenced by aversion can lead to labeling everything as either good or bad and can manifest as believing a certain group of people are good while others are bad. This results in disharmony with others who do not share the same view, in extreme case this leads to discrimination and can even lead to fights or war.

Abhinivesha, desire for life, an intensive will to live or fear of death. Abhinivesha also includes the incorrect identification of the true self with the temporary physical body, blocking attainment of enlightenment and liberation. Patanjali describes abhinivesha as the source of stopping spiritual growth. Yoga practices of asana, pranayama and meditation are methods to overcome abhinivesha.

KOSHAS: 5 SHEATHS

1. Annamaya Kosha.
2. Pranamaya Kosha.
3. Manomaya Kosha.
4. Vijanamaya Kosha.
5. Anandamaya Kosha.

The koshas are sheaths or energy layers that start from the outer layer of the skin to our deep spiritual core.

Annamaya kosha represents the physical body including the skin, muscles, connective tissue, fat and bones and is nourished by food.

Pranamaya kosha represents the subtle or pranic body, it is the circulation system for Prana and includes the blood, lymph and cardiovascular system.

Manomaya kosha takes us deep into the mind, emotions, nervous system and sensory organs. It is responsible for controlling the messages sent from the brain to the nervous system.

Vijanamaya kosha is the intellectual sheath where we develop awareness, insight, consciousness and discrimination.

Anandamaya kosha is composed of bliss and is a true reflection of Atman, the soul.

NADIS - ENERGY CHANNELS

The human body is made up of many energy channels called Nadis. The ancient yogis with their divine vision were able to visualize and identify 72,000 Nadis, the names and descriptions are seen in texts on tantra and yoga.

The 3 main Nadis are Ida, Pingala and Sushumna, which play an important part in our pranayama practice, Ida is identified with breaths of the left nostril and Pingala is identified with breaths of the right. As far as energy is concerned left is represented by lunar energy and called Chandra Nadi, right is represented by solar energy and is called Surya Nadi. These two Nadis start at the coccyx region and rise upwards in an encircled manner to reach the top. Sushumna Nadi is in the middle and runs between Ida and Pingala.

PRANA

Prana translates as vital life force. In China it is called Chi or Qi. In yoga we call this energy prana. The universe consists of prana, in our body prana flows through the energy pathways called nadis.

VAYUS

Five types of prana collectively known as vayu's are referred to in Hindu texts. Prana Vayu is considered the most important and all the others arise from it.

1. Prana Vayu.
2. Apana Vayu.
3. Udana Vayu.
4. Samana Vayu.
5. Vyana Vayu.

Prana Vayu refers to the breath responsible for nourishing our whole bodily system, it is situated in the lungs.

Apana Vayu refers to down and outward energy of the eliminatory system, it is situated in the hips and gut.

Udana Vayu refers to rising energy, it is situated in the throat and is responsible for sound, speaking, crying and laughing.

Samana Vayu refers to the heat of digestion, it is situated in the stomach.

Vyana Vayu refers to the energy of circulation, it is situated throughout the body.

CHAKRAS - ENERGY CENTRES

Chakras are centers of subtle vital energy in the sushumna nadi. They are storage centers for consciousness and energy. The chakras have corresponding centers in the gross physical body, each one represents a state of consciousness and have a specific feeling of bliss or joy. The 7 chakras are located at the base of the spine to the top of the head.

1. Muladhara chakra
2. Swadhisthana chakra
3. Manipura chakra
4. Anahata chakra
5. Vishuddha chakra
6. Ajna chakra
7. Sahasrara chakra

Muladhara chakra is located at the base of the spine and is often called the 'root chakra' and corresponds to the sacral plexus. It is connected to the earth element, its color is red and is associated with the sound 'Lam'. This is also said to be where Kundalini rests.

Swadhisthana chakra is located in the pelvic region, relates to the sexual organs and corresponds to the prostrate plexus. It is connected to the water element, its color is orange and is associated with the sound 'Vam'

Manipura chakra is located at the naval region, relates to the digestive system and corresponds to the solar plexus. It is connected to the fire element, its color is yellow and is associated with the sound 'Ram'.

Anahata chakra is located in the heart region, relates to our emotions and corresponds to the cardiac plexus. It is connected to the air element, its color is green and is associated with the sound 'Yam'.

Vishuddha chakra is located in the throat region and corresponds to the laryngeal plexus. It is connected to the ether element, its color is blue and is associated by the sound 'Ham'.

Ajna chakra is located between the eyebrows or the third eye in front of the brain. It relates to our intuition, visualization and imagination, and corresponds to the cavernous plexus, it is connected to the ether element, its color is purple and is associated with the sound 'Om'.

Sahasrara chakra is located at the crown of the head. It transcends all of the elements, colors and sounds. When it is balanced we are connected to the source of all life.

KRIYAS - CLEANSING PROCESSES

In Hinduism there are six Kriyas that should be practiced to maintain good health.

1. Navali (Nauli)
2. Neti.
3. Dhouti.
4. Basti.
5. Kapalbhati.
6. Trataka.

Nauli Kriya is the practice of moving the abdominal muscles, this stimulates and cures all problems in the intestines, colon and other organs of the digestive system.

Procedure: stand with legs apart, knees bent slightly, place your hands just above the knees, bend forward a little, exhale then draw in the stomach.

You create a column like structure in the central abdominal muscles, be in this position for a short time then release the muscles and breathe normally, this is

Madhyama nauli. With practice you can move the central column to the left and right, to the left is called Vama Nauli to the right is called Dakshina Nauli.

Neti Kriya clears the nasal tract, a special container called a 'neti pot' is used.

Procedure: fill the neti pot with luke warm saline water. Stand with the legs a little apart, bend forward slightly with the mouth open, turn the head to the right, insert the tip of the neti pot into the left nostril, the water comes in through the left nostril and drains out of the right nostril, repeat the procedure with the opposite nostril. When you are finished squeeze the nose gently to remove any excess water.

Dhouti Kriya cleanses the digestive tract from the throat to the stomach, a cotton strip or ribbon about one metre in length is used.

Procedure: stand or sit in a comfortable posture with the back straight and start swallowing the ribbon keeping hold of the other end of the ribbon. After a short time slowly draw out the ribbon, the toxins and bile will come out with the ribbon. After a couple of hours you can eat soft non-spicy liquid food.

Basti Kriya stimulates and cleanses the anal passage and rectum.

Procedure: sit in a bathtub and start drawing water in through the anus by repeatedly contracting and relaxing the sphincter muscles. Through this action water fills the rectum and lower part of the colon, after some time the water with residual toxins comes out. In the west we call this colonic cleansing, where a rubber tube is inserted into the anus and water is gravity fed into the rectum.

Kapalbhati Kriya is a pranayama technique that stimulates and strengthens the lungs.

Procedure: sit in a comfortable posture with the back straight, inhale fully then, with force, exhale by drawing in the stomach, repeat the exhalations quickly, inhalation will be passive and happen automatically, just concentrate on the exhalation. 50 to 100 exhalations repeated five times is a recommended practice.

Trataka Kriya improves clarity of vision by strengthening the eye muscles.

Procedure: sit in a comfortable position with the back straight, place a candle in front of you at a safe distance. Look into the flame of the candle and try not to blink, the eyes will start to water cleansing the eyes. After some time close the eyes and place the fingertips lightly on the eyelids giving a slow gentle massage, then open the eyes slowly.

FOUR PATHS OF YOGA

1. Karma Yoga - yoga of action.
2. Bhakti Yoga - yoga of devotion.
3. Raja Yoga - yoga of mind control.
4. Jnana Yoga – yoga of knowledge.

Karma Yoga is dedication of all work and actions as an offering to the supreme with no thought of personal gain 'all work is Gods work'. By giving up the rewards of one's action, the action becomes un-selfish. By not concentrating on your personal needs or desires and by trying to help everyone, including humans, animals and the whole world our heart opens, the ego is destroyed and oneness is attained. Karma yoga can be practiced at all times.

Bhakti Yoga is the devotional approach of pure love, Bhakti is said to be the safest and easiest form of yoga to practice by channeling the emotions towards devotion. Prayer, chanting mantra, study of religious texts and puja ceremonies are the basic methods. Bhakti yoga frees the individual of emotions and ego by developing humility and surrender to the supreme.

Raja Yoga means the royal path, just as a king needs to maintain control of his kingdom the raja yogi maintains control over the mind by using yoga practices of meditation, pranayama and asana. The divine self is clouded by disturbances of the mind, if the body and mind can be made pure, settled and at ease the inner self will shine through.

Jnana Yoga is the path of knowledge, the intellectual approach to attain enlightenment. Through self-analysis, reason and discrimination the mind is used to examine its own nature. Jnana yoga is said to be the most difficult because it uses the mind and intellect to go beyond yourself to realize you are one with the divine. Jnana yoga is the study of ancient texts of Vedanta philosophy to learn to discriminate what is real and unreal, what is true and untrue through study and self-inquiry. Vedanta says that liberation cannot be gained by ritual, action, duty or charity, only through personal intuitive experience. Ramana Maharishi the Indian saint when asked would often reply "first ask yourself who is asking the question"

AYURVEDA - TRADITIONAL INDIAN MEDICINE

Ayurveda translates as 'the science of life' it is said to be over 5,000 years old the same as traditional Chinese medicine TCM. It is the traditional healing system of India, modern western medicine is only 2,000 ears old. Ayurveda is a combination of mind, body energy and spirit. Its purpose is to heal, cure and maintain quality of life, where modern western medicine only aims to suppress symptoms of disease. According to Ayurveda everyone is unique and treatments should be customized to each individual, modern western medicine takes the approach of one treatments fits all. Ayurveda deals with the symptoms to get to the root cause of disease, it includes diet and nutrition, lifestyle, medicinal herbs, exercise, breathing meditation and healing treatments. The body's energy 'Prana' is the foundation of everything we do, it should be strong, vibrant and supple. The five senses, hearing, smell, taste, sight and touch are how we interact with the outside world, they should be clear and sharp. The mind is the home to our consciousness, it should be calm, centered and balanced. The heart is the home our soul, it should be open, free from anger and resentment.

DOSHAS - BODY TYPES

In Ayurveda the whole universe is an interplay of the energies of the 5 elements, ayurveda groups the elements into 3 basic body types, When they are in balance they support life, when they are not, life is in disharmony. Each person is born with a unique constitution with a leading and secondary dosha.

1. Vata - Air and Ether.
2. Pitta -Fire and Water.
3. Kapha - Water and Earth.

Vata is associated with movement and controls breathing, blinking and heart beat. People who are vata tend to be thinner, taller, faster, quick thinking, creative and flexible. When out of balance they are unstable, anxious and fearing which can result in poor digestion, insomnia and psychological problems.

Pitta is associated with metabolism and digestion. People who are pitta tend to be medium build, muscular, balanced, out going and are usually decision makers. When unbalanced they can be hot headed, angry and hostile, which can result in high blood pressure, heart disease and inflammatory disorders.

Kapha is associated with structure and balance of fluids in the body. People who are kapha tend to be heavier, large boned, balanced, stable, calm, loving and forgiving. When unbalanced they can be overly attached, insecure, possessive and greedy which can result in congestion, respiratory problems and obesity.

FIVE ELEMENTS

1. Earth
2. Water
3. Fire
4. Air
5. Ether - space

In western culture only four elements are recognized, earth, water, fire and air, in the east a fifth element is recognized, ether / space.

GUNAS - SUBTLE QUALITIES

The three gunas underlie all of creation, as the dosha represent body types, the gunas represent mind types, both on the surface and deep within our consciousness. The gunas also relate to food.

1. Tamas - dark, lazy
2. Rajas - energy
3. Sattva - pure

Tamas is characterized by inertia, stagnation, lack of movement, dullness, darkness, and heaviness that creates ignorance, stifles change and transformation.

Tamasik food is old, stale, toxic, and sour, which creates inactivity and sickness.

Rajas is characterized by motion, evolution, growth, desire, craving success and lack of integrity.

Rajasik food is highly spiced, too hot or too cold, which creates hyper activity and anger.

Sattva is characterized by balance, harmony, stability, clarity, happiness, contentment and good energy.

Sattvik food is normal, easy to digest, fresh, nutritious and balanced.

BE THE CHANGE.

Throughout our lives we are constantly drawn to what is external to us. This has created a strong program in our minds that makes us think we are happier if changes happen in line with our expectations or desires.

Were you ever able to remain permanently happy by anything that happened in your life? If any change outside made you happy, how long did it last? When another change happens it brings another feeling, this could be happy or sad.

The whole of our life is a continuing process depending on outside change. At some point in our life we have to stop and think about this fact and make a new start in which 'you can be the change' this means you are ready to enter the path of self reflection.

'To be the change' is the first step to experience your true potential in life.

Since we do not have control of changes happening on the outside, it always has the chance of bringing sorrow or unhappiness. When you are in the state of 'be the change' you have the ability to gain control and be more able to live a harmonious life.

When you introduce yoga into your daily life you will be starting the process of 'be the change' in your deeper self.

Many people miss the chance to 'be the change' because the ego fights this and the chance to 'be the change' is lost.

When you are driving and if someone obstructs your way you might immediately get upset without thinking, building negative emotions in yourself, this is the mind focusing on the negative, it is your reaction that makes you upset, you have the choice to react of not react, by not reacting you will not allow yourself to get upset.

THOUGHTS

When you look at your thought process, what is it? Why do you have thoughts? How many thoughts do you have in a day? Are thoughts real or unreal?

It is not easy to be thoughtless due to the conditioning of the mind, what is this conditioning? It is nothing more than holding onto what has already passed or projecting what is likely to happen in the future. Conditioning of the mind means you are not living life in the present, yet paradoxically life can only be in the present. To live in the present is to live in the real life beyond thoughts.

Due to these uncontrolled fluctuations of the mind your true self has no space to express itself. Only when you are able to control the fluctuations of the mind your true self is expressed, with true awareness, this is the path of yoga and you move from egotistical thoughts toward the Divine self with awareness of existence.

Patanjali says in his second sutra (PYS 1.2)

"Citta Vrithi Nirodahah" "Yoga is controlling the fluctuations of the mind"

SECTION 11: DIET, VITAMINS, MINERALS, PROTEINS, FATS

In my previous book 'Yoga and Diet cured my arthritis' I gave advice on diet and how processed food, food in packets, tins and fast foods which contain, preservatives, colorings, taste enhancers, E numbers etc are responsible for creating diseases such as arthritis, diabetes, heart disease and cancers, I feel this is so important to everyone so I am repeating parts of it here. We are seeing a worldwide increase in the above diseases that is directly related to the commercial food industry. This industry is largely unregulated and chemical additives are not tested for their negative effects on our system. Medicinal drugs are extensively tested before they are released on to the market, this is not the case with food additives.

I am not going to ask anyone to be vegetarian or non-vegetarian, I think the human body can benefit from meat products especially organ meats and fish, which I include on the following lists. Some people need meat; some people don't. From a yoga point of view a vegetarian diet may make you more flexible but if you lack strength this can also be a hindrance.

If you do choose meat, try to get organic meat from your local farm store, farmer's market or the organic section at your supermarket. Too many growth hormones and antibiotics are randomly used in the commercial food chain, especially in the innocent chicken which is pumped full of antibiotics and growth hormones to meet the demands of the increasing market.

You need to feed your body with the nutrients and vitamins it requires by eating the correct seasonal foods that are organically produced wherever possible. Too often our bodies do not absorb sufficient nutrients due to the chemicals, additives, colourings, and preservatives in our daily food

Get into the habit of reading the information on packaged food to identify the contents. For example, fruit yoghurt may contain white sugar or artificial sweeteners even though it says organic and natural on the front! The packaging will also identify E numbers, chemical preservatives and colourings. As a rule of thumb the longer the list of 'things' in packaged foods the more likely it is to be a problem in terms of additives, lack of freshness and actual nutrition.

BENEFICIAL VITAMIN, MINERAL, PROTEIN AND FAT SOURCES

In this section I list our essential nutrients and the benefits they have for our system. I then list the foods that contain the nutrients we require. Many of the foods appear several times and on different lists, showing how easy it is to choose and eat a healthy balanced diet.

VITAMINS.

VITAMIN A

Deficiency can cause defects in bone formation, vitamin A strengthens our immune system making us resistant to infection.

Best foods:

- Spinach,
- Bok choi,
- Sweet potato,
- Apple cider vinegar,
- Carrots,
- Mustard leaf,
- Turnip leaf,
- Beet leaf,
- Kale,
- Swiss chard,
- Winter squash,
- Broccoli,
- Yoghurt,
- Calf liver,
- Millet,
- Eggs - free range,
- Bananas,
- Sesame seeds,
- Sunflower seeds,
- Raisins,
- Raw vegetables.

VITAMIN B (THIAMINE)

Lack of vitamin B can cause loss of muscle tone, depression, anaemia, fatigue, constipation and decreased fertility.

Best foods:

- Red meat, beef heart, kidneys, liver
- Oily fish e.g. mackerel,
- Free range eggs,
- Cheese,
- Soya,
- Crab (can be bad for gout),
- Brewers yeast.

VITAMIN B2 (RIBOFLAVIN)

Is beneficial to the soft tissues of the body,

Lack of Vitamin B2 can cause nervous depression, fatigue, confusion, dermatitis and eye problems.

Best foods:

- Cheese,
- Almonds,
- Red meat,
- Free range egg,

- Mushroom,
- Sesame seeds,
- Spinach,
- Squid,

- Oily fish,

- Raw milk.

VITAMIN B5 (PANTOTHENIC ACID)

Good for liver function helps the brain and nervous system. Prevents fatigue and muscle cramps.

Best foods:

- Mushrooms,
- Cheese,
- Avocado,

- Eggs,
- Sweet potatoes
- Sunflower seeds,

- Fish,
- Free-range chicken,
- Liver.

VITAMIN B6 (PYRIDOXINE)

Regulates red blood cell metabolism along the nervous and immune systems, lack of can lead to depression and increase risk of heart attack.

Best foods:

- Sunflower seeds,
- Pistachio nuts,
- Tuna,

- Free range chicken and turkey,
- Dried prunes,

- Bananas,
- Avocados,
- Leafy greens.

VITAMIN B12 (COBALAMIN)

Deficiency can lead to anaemia, fatigue and depression. Long-term deficiency can cause permanent damage to the brain and nervous system.

Best foods:

- Oily fish,
- Crab,
- Liver,
- Tofu,
- All bran,
- Organic milk,
- Swiss cheese,
- Free range eggs.

VITAMIN C (ASCORBIC ACID)

Can be used in high doses against colds and infections and is a powerful antioxidant. The body requires it to maintain healthy blood vessels, cartilage and production of collagen.

Best foods:

- Bell pepper - yellow, red, or green,
- Guava,
- Leafy vegetables,
- Kale,
- Kiwi fruit,
- Broccoli,
- Strawberries,
- Oranges,
- Tomato,
- Papaya,
- Peas,
- Grapes,
- Gooseberry,
- Citrus fruits.

VITAMIN D

Essential for all arthritis sufferers, as the body needs it to absorb calcium and phosphorous from foods for bone development, immune functioning and alleviation of inflammation, deficiency can increase the risk of cancer, poor hair growth and Osteomalacia. One of the best ways of absorbing Vitamin D is sunshine.

Best foods:

- Cod liver oil,
- Oily fish,
- Apple
- Mushrooms,
- Tofu,
- Caviar,
- Organic milk,
- Lean pork
- Free range eggs,

- Almond milk,
- Soya milk,
- Bananas
- Sesame seeds
- Sunflower seeds.

VITAMIN E

Helps prevent against heart disease, cancer and eye disease. Aids proper liver functioning and promotes radiant hair and skin.

Best foods:

- Leafy vegetables,
- Spinach,
- Almonds,
- Sunflower seeds,
- Avocado,
- Shrimps,
- Salmon,
- Trout,
- Olive oil,
- Broccoli,
- Squash pumpkin,
- Kiwi fruit,
- Free range eggs.

VITAMIN F

Unsaturated fatty acids

Important in the repair and development of tissues, wound healing, hair growth and reproductive system.

Best foods:

- Oils - peanut, safflower, sunflower, soy, walnut,
- Nuts and seeds,
- Oily fish,
- Tofu,
- Fresh vegetables.

VITAMIN K

Essential vitamin against blood clotting can treat Osteoporosis and Alzheimer's disease and helps prevent cancer and heart disease.

- Best foods:
- Herbs,
- Leafy vegetables, kale, spinach,
- Spring onions,
- Chilies,
- Asparagus,
- Cucumber,
- Cooked soya beans,
- Olive oil,

- Dried fruit,
- Figs,
- Liver.
- Prunes,
- Tomatoes,
- Blueberries,
- Egg yolk,

VITAMIN P (BIOFLAVANOIDS - RELATED TO VITAMIN C)

Help maintain healthy blood vessels, veins and capillaries.

Best foods:

- Plant based food,
- Leafy greens, spinach,
- Watercress.
- Citrus fruits,
- Green peppers,

Notice how a lot of the same foods show up on the above lists, we do not need vitamin supplements if the food we are consuming is rich in nutrients. A lot of the same vitamins are helpful for bone and muscle health and for stopping inflammation. They are essential for arthritis sufferers.

You will also notice the same with the following list of minerals, we can eat our way to good health, enjoy all the fresh choices available, food should be enjoyed 'eat for health'.

We all react differently to certain foods, keep a diary and exclude the foods that cause any reaction, slowly add new foods so you can gauge the reaction on your system.

MINERALS

CALCIUM

Essential mineral for arthritis sufferers as it helps to build strong bones and teeth. It regulates muscle contractions including heartbeat.

Best foods:

- Green vegetables,
- Farm chicken,
- Tofu,
- Seafood,
- Cheese,
- Sardines,
- Liver,
- Dairy products,
- Free range eggs,
- French beans,
- Pilchards.

IRON

Helps the blood carry oxygen to the cells and to remove carbon dioxide.

Best foods:

- Leafy greens,
- Liver,
- Free range eggs,
- Beans,
- Nuts,
- Dried fruit,
- Whole grains,
- Brown rice.

PHOSPHORUS

Essential for proper functioning of nerves, glands, muscles and bone formation

Best foods:

- Meat,
- Fish,
- Free range eggs,
- Farm chicken,
- Nuts,
- Sunflower seeds,
- Broccoli,
- Peas.

MAGNESIUM

Activates enzymes.

Best foods:

- Brewers yeast,
- Leafy greens,
- Oily fish, mackerel,
- Almonds,
- Wheat Bran,
- Cocoa,
- Cashews,
- Pumpkin seeds.

COPPER

Essential for bone and connective tissue production, deficiency leads to osteoporosis, joint pain and lowered immunity.

Best foods:

- Seafood,
- Leafy greens,
- Mushrooms,
- Seeds,
- Nuts,
- Beans pulses,

- Dried fruit,
- Avocados,
- Goat's cheese,
- Brown rice,
- Soya,
- Fermented tofu,
- Tempeh,
- Miso.

POTASSIUM

Aids a proper digestive system, feeds the heart, kidney and muscles.

Best foods:

- Leafy greens,
- Bananas,
- Summer squash,
- Mushrooms,
- Yogurt,
- Oily fish,
- Fruits,
- Berries,
- Apple cider vinegar.

IODINE

Regulates the metabolism through the thyroid.

Best foods:

- Fish,
- Shellfish,
- Organic cereals and grains.

"Again we see a lot of the same foods coming up".

Remember when you buy food, try to get organic or locally produced seasonal fruits, vegetables, whole grains and meat. When cooking do not use too much water and do not cook for too long, the closer to raw the more nutrients remain. DO NOT throw away any cooking water, save it and add it to your smoothies, juices or soups. Steaming is a great way to prepare fresh vegetables, no more cans or jars. Take your time and enjoy the process, knowing you are actually feeding yourself to maintain health.

PROTEINS

Proteins, made up mainly of amino acids, are our basic requirement, they are essential for our tissues, muscles, organs, blood and all the cells in our body.

Arthritis sufferers have to be extremely aware as protein deficiency can lead to severe attacks. Look out for early signs: lack of energy, fatigue, irregular bowel movements, constipation, swelling and increase in body weight.

Best Foods:

- Muscle meat, e.g. steaks
- Kidneys, liver,
- Farm chicken,
- Fish,
- Seafood,
- Raw milk,
- Yoghurt,
- Farm eggs,
- Cheese,
- Cottage cheese,
- Tofu,
- Soya beans,
- Seeds and nuts,
- Green beans,
- Beans and legumes,
- Cacao,
- Sprouted beans.

ESSENTIAL AMINO ACIDS.

Daily intake can be obtained by mixing one-part pulses with two parts brown rice or millet. It is a great carbohydrate and protein mix for your new diet.

FATS AND OILS

Most of our body's fat requirement is taken from vegetable oils and some meats, fish, cheese, nuts, seeds, raw milk and yogurt.

Fats can have a bad image; people think if they eat fats or oils they are going to get fat but this is not necessarily the case. Our body needs fat as part of a controlled diet. High consumption of saturated fats has been shown to effect cardiac health. Likewise trans fats, often created by high cooking temperatures and deep-frying, have been linked with certain types of cancer and should be limited in the diet, so we need to be careful to use the right fats, oils and cooking methods. Cold pressed oils retain more nutrition than other oils and fats.

Best foods:

- Cold pressed olive oil for salads and cooking is the best choice along with sunflower, peanut, sesame oil.
- Fatty cuts of meat,
- Butter,
- Ghee, (clarified butter).
- Cheese, especially hard cheese,
- Cream, soured cream,
- Some savoury snacks and chocolate,
- Coconut oil.

CARBOHYDRATES

Carbohydrates provide fuel for the body.

Best foods:

- Fruits,
- Sweet potato,
- Quinoa,
- Millet,
- Beans, légumes, lentils,
- Grains,
- Seeds,
- Oats,
- Couscous,
- Carrot,
- Buckwheat,
- Brown rice,
- Cereals,
- Noodles (no wheat),
- Free range eggs,
- Dairy,
- Dried fruits,
- Honey,
- Molasses,
- Nuts and nut butter,
- Fruit juice.

Get your carbohydrates from these natural foods that will also give you the added benefit of vitamins and minerals. Stay away from the refined over-processed carbohydrates in cakes, ice cream, candy, jams, crisps, bread, white rice, spaghetti and most processed foods.

Our system is not designed to take on the extra burden of trying to break down chemicals that have little or no nutritional value and are put in to food to make it last longer, look brighter, and taste sweeter.

Eating too much refined sugar, wheat, rice and other grains can lead to fatigue, because the system is overloaded from refined foods blocking and over-working it.

OMEGA 3 FATTY ACIDS

Help prevent inflammation and decrease symptoms of arthritis.

Best foods:

- Salmon,
- Herrings,
- Sardines,
- Trout,
- Mackerel,
- Oysters,
- Squid,
- Flax seeds,
- Walnuts,
- Chia seeds,
- Fish roe,
- Caviar,
- Soya beans,
- Tofu,
- Spinach,
- Winter squash,
- Kale,
- Broccoli,
- Olive oil,
- Flaxseed oil,
- Canola oil.

- Cod liver oil.

TOP 10 RAW FOODS

We hear a lot about 'super' foods these days and sometimes what is in fashion can also carry a price tag to match. There are all types of cost effective alternatives out there, you have to learn to be your own nutritionist.

- Coconut,

- Chia seeds,

- Leafy greens,

- Seeds,

- Seaweed,

- Sprouts,

- Blueberries,

- Bee pollen,

- Raw chocolate,

- Cacao nibs.

APPENDIX 1: GLOSSARY OF TERMS

This glossary contains terms and concepts used in this document. Many Hindu and Sanskrit words and concepts are explained in detail in the text and are not included here.

Unless otherwise stated definitions and explanations are sourced from the Oxford online dictionary https://en.oxforddictionaries.com..

Asana: From Sanskrit āsana seat, manner of sitting. A posture adopted in performing hatha yoga.

Ashtanga yoga (astanga): A type of yoga based on eight principles and consisting of a series of poses executed in swift succession, vinyasa, combined with deep, controlled breathing, bandha body locks and Dristhi gazing point.

From Hindi aṣṭaṇ or its source, Sanskrit ashṭaṅga having eight parts, from ashtán eight.

Aum, Ohm, Om.: A mystic syllable, considered the most sacred mantra in Hinduism and Tibetan Buddhism. It appears at the beginning and end of most Sanskrit recitations, prayers, and texts.

Ayurveda/Ayurvedic: The traditional Hindu system of medicine, which is based on the idea of balance in bodily systems and uses diet, herbal treatment, and yogic breathing.

Bandha: Body lock (in yoga).

Carbohydrate: Any of a large group of organic compounds occurring in foods and living tissues and including sugars, starch, and cellulose. They can be broken down to release energy in the body.

Cartilage: Firm, flexible connective tissue found in various forms in the larynx and respiratory tract, in structures such as the external ear, and in the articulating surfaces of joints.

Cervical spine: The neck.

Circulation: The continuous motion by which the blood travels through all parts of the body under the action of the heart.

Dristhi: Gazing point (in yoga).

E numbers: E numbers are codes for substances that are permitted for use as food additives within the European Union and other jurisdictions. For more information and the list of E numbers: https://en.wikipedia.org/wiki/E_number

Glaucoma: A common eye condition in which the fluid pressure inside the eye rises to a level higher than healthy for that eye.

Growth hormone: A hormone that stimulates growth in animal or plant cells, especially (in animals) that is secreted by the pituitary gland.

Guru: A Hindu spiritual teacher.

Hatha yoga: The branch of yoga which concentrates on physical health and mental well-being through postures (asanas), breathing techniques (pranayama), and meditation (dyana) http://medical-dictionary.thefreedictionary.com/hatha+yoga

Hatha Yoga Pradipika: The Hatha Yoga Pradīpikā) is a classic Sanskrit manual on hatha yoga, written by Svāmi Svātmārāma, a disciple of Swami Gorakhnath in the 15th Century. https://en.wikipedia.org/wiki/Hatha_Yoga_Pradipika

Hormones: A chemical substance produced in the body that controls and regulates the activity of certain cells or organs. Hormones are essential for every activity of life, including the processes of digestion, metabolism, growth, reproduction, and mood control. Many hormones, such as neurotransmitters, are active in more than one physical process.

Immune system: A complex system that is responsible for distinguishing a person from everything foreign to him or her and for protecting the body against infections and foreign substances.

Iyengar yoga/BKS Iyengar: A type of Hatha yoga focusing on the correct alignment of the body, making use of straps, wooden blocks, and other objects as aids in achieving the correct postures. BKS Iyengar was also a student of Krishnamacharya.

Jumping back and through: See Vinyassa

Karma: In Hinduism and Buddhism the sum of a person's actions in this and previous states of existence, viewed as deciding their fate in future existences.

Meditate: To focus one's mind for a period of time, in silence or with the aid of chanting, for religious or spiritual purposes or as a method of relaxation.

Mineral: An inorganic substance needed by the human body for good health.

Mindfulness: A mental state achieved by focusing one's awareness on the present moment, while calmly acknowledging and accepting one's feelings, thoughts, and bodily sensations, used as a therapeutic technique.

Mudra: A symbolic or ritual hand gesture.

Nutrient, nutritious, nourishing: A substance that provides nourishment essential for the maintenance of life and for growth.

Omega 3 fatty acid: An unsaturated fatty acid occurring chiefly in fish oils.

Organic: Of food or farming methods produced or involving production without the use of chemical fertilizers, pesticides, or other artificial chemicals.

Plexus: A network of nerves in the body.

Prana: Lifeforce, Chi, Qi

Pranayama: In yoga, the conscious and careful regulation of breath.

Processed foods: The term 'processed food' applies to any food that has been altered from its natural state in some way, either for safety reasons or convenience. Food processing techniques include freezing, canning, baking, drying and pasteurising products. http://www.nhs.uk/Livewell/Goodfood/Pages/what-are-processed-foods.aspx For more info see

http://www.eatright.org/resource/food/nutrition/nutrition-facts-and-food-labels/avoiding-processed-foods

Protein: Nitrogenous organic compounds which are an essential part of all living organisms, especially as structural components of body tissues such as muscle, hair, etc., and as enzymes and antibodies.

Refined grains: Refining grains removes varying proportions of the bran and germ. Because micronutrients are generally present in higher concentrations in these outer layers of the grain, refined grain products are lower in vitamins and minerals than whole grains. For more information see: http://www.glnc.org.au/grains/grains-and-nutrition/refined-grains/

Repetitive stress syndrome or injury: An injury that occurs due to recurrent overuse or improper use of a limb or joint.

Restrict: Put a limit on; keep under control.

Samadhi: A state of enlightenment achieved through meditation.

Stress: A state of mental or emotional strain or tension resulting from adverse or demanding circumstances.

Supplement: A thing added to something else in order to complete or enhance it.

Surya Namaskar: Sun salutation

Ujayi breath: Breathing with sound (in ashtanga yoga).

Vinyasa: A vinyasa, in essence, consists of moving from one asana, or body position, to another, combining breathing with the movement. The Surya Namaskar and each of the successive asanas are comprised of a particular number of vinyasas.

Vitamin: Any of a group of organic compounds that are essential for normal growth and nutrition and are required in small quantities in the diet because they cannot be synthesized by the body.

Whole grain: Describes an intact grain, flour or a food that contains all three parts of the grain. For more information see: http://www.glnc.org.au/grains/grains-and-nutrition/wholegrains/

Yoga: Yoga is a group of physical, mental, and spiritual practices or disciplines that originated in ancient India. There is a broad variety of Yoga schools, practices, and goals. In Vedic Sanskrit, yoga (from the root yuj) means "to add", "to join", "to unite", or "to attach" in its most common literal sense.

Yogi, yogin, yogini: Someone who practices yoga or follows the yoga philosophy with a high level of commitment. https://en.wikipedia.org/wiki/Yoga

AUTHOR BIO

Mark Flint was diagnosed with rheumatoid arthritis over 25 years ago. He had always been fit and athletic, an ex-professional golfer and successful businessman. When diagnosed he was advised to take a steroid a day for the rest of his life or end up in a wheelchair. He chose not to take this advice. Instead, he went on a course of discovery about how to put his body back together without resorting to medications. He began by experimenting with foods to find an arthritis friendly diet and trying various other alternative remedies and treatments.

Born and raised in the UK Mark now lives in Mysore India with his wife Stephanie and young son Oliver. There they run a heritage guesthouse 'Shanti Nilayam' have a business making yoga accessories and also teach yoga around Asia for several months each year. It is in Mysore that Mark discovered the benefits of a regular yoga practice to his condition. He began practicing yoga in 1999 and later moved on to the ashtanga yoga system under the guidance of Sharath and Saraswathi Jois in 2009. In 2012 Mark was authorised by the K. Pattabhi Jois Ashtanga Institute to teach this style of traditional ashtanga yoga, and is also Yoga Alliance ERYT 500 (experienced yoga teacher) and owner of Parampara YA registred yoga school.

After the COVID 19 Pandemic that has taken its grip on all aspects of everyone's lives in 2020, Mark as made a decision to leave his beloved Mysore behind and relocate to the Algarve in Southern Portugal with his family in early 2021.

Sharing yoga will remain his main priority with online classes, tutorials, Yoga alliance online teacher trainings, and private classes whilst searching for land to build a yoga retreat and training centre. See MARKFLINTYOGA.ORG for further information.

International yoga conferences, workshops and Teacher training's will resume as travel permits.

WWW. MARKFLINTYOGA.ORG

www.ingramcontent.com/pod-product-compliance
Lightning Source LLC
Chambersburg PA
CBHW080558030426
42336CB00019B/3238